"I have long recommended the work of John Sarno, and his mind-body approach to chronic pain. As a student and colleague of Sarno, Dr. Schechter is able to explain the mechanism involved and tell you not only *what* to think about pain, but challenge you to explore *how* to think about pain in order to get relief."

> Andrew Weil, M.D.
> Author of *8 Weeks to Optimum Health* and *Healthy Aging*

"I highly recommend Dr. Schechter's book. It is readable, accessible, and insightful, and based on his long history in the diagnosis and treatment of Tension Myoneural Syndrome (TMS)."

> John E. Sarno, M.D.
> Professor of Rehabilitation Medicine
> NYU School of Medicine

"Chronic low back pain is more likely a brain than a back disorder. Dr. Schechter's focus on the brain and the cognitive retraining he offers patients has proven value in treatment. Dr. Schechter's clinical evaluations of the cognitive and psychosocial issues are astute and this book focuses on the symbiosis between mental health and chronic pain."

> Thomas Jones, M.D.
> Neurosurgeon and Medical Director
> Santa Barbara Neuroscience Institute

"Dr. David Schechter is one of the most skilled and experienced physicians in the entire country in the treatment of chronic pain with a mind-body approach (TMS). Not only has he helped dozens of my patients in their recovery, he played a significant role in the elimination of my own chronic pain symptoms."

> Alan Gordon, LCSW
> Director of the Pain Psychology Center
> USC School of Social Work.

Praise from Physicians, Therapists and Practitioners

"Dr. David Schechter has written a book derived from years of medical experience--full of human wisdom, compassion and excellent practical guidance for those who suffer from chronic and unexplained pain. The book allows the reader an enlightening conversation with a man who not only is an expert in mind-body treatment, but who cares enough about his patients to want to save them unnecessary suffering, time, detrimental procedures and costs. A clarifying contribution to this otherwise confusing and painful subject."

Arnold Chanon Bloch, LCSW
Psychotherapist.

"*Think Away Your Pain*" has advanced Mind Body Medicine to a whole new level! Dr. David Schechter's vast knowledge and effectiveness in teaching those with chronic pain to control their own destiny through self-awareness has allowed his patients to become independent and often pain-free. The philosophy and methodology of "*Think Away Your Pain*" is a life changer!"

Matthew Stodolsky, PT, MSPT
Physical Therapist

"If you are in chronic pain or know someone that is, this is an important book. Dr. Schechter's book is a beacon of light on the long, dark, chronic pain journey. With his compassionate insight, and formidable experience, Dr. Schechter teaches us how we can focus on the psychological rather than get caught up in our physical symptoms. This is the key to recovery. He teaches us how we can actually think away our pain..."

Jill Solomon, MFT
Psychotherapist

"In *Think Away Your Pain*, Dr. David Schechter truly demystifies the concept of mind-body pain, and provides clear and concrete steps that pain sufferers can take to finally heal their pain. This book is an ideal resource for pain sufferers and healing professionals alike."

Jessica Oifer, MA
Marriage and Family Therapist

Testimonials from Actual Patients and Professionals

"Dr. David Schechter's book is a watershed event; for those who have suffered for years this comprehensive assault on inexplicable pain is a torch in the darkness to lead the sufferer back to a pain-free, joyous existence. The genuineness of the man is reflected in the text; I know because I suffered in the prison of my body for 27 years until he worked with me and set me free."

David Shapiro, Film/TV Composer

"Dr. Schechter has been able to write about TMS and the connection between my brain and pain in a way that I could easily understand, relate to and apply in my daily life. With Dr. Schechter's book and guidance, I came to appreciate how the many doctors that came before him actually perpetuated my symptoms and reinforced a mindset of frailty within me. The role that physical pain plays in my life has greatly diminished since I've read his work and in those rare instances where pain tries to creep in, I have a consolidated and clear resource that I quickly turn to as my line of first defense. For this, I am grateful!"

John Sutton, Vice President
Fortune 500 Company

"I was introduced to Dr. Schechter a couple of years ago through Dr. John Sarno's office at NYU. I was at my wit's end, suffering from debilitating headaches. I could not work, let alone sleep or even eat. Nothing seemed to help, and I was ultimately advised by specialists that I would need to take powerful medication with severe side-effects for probably the rest of my life. Probably the most important gift he gave me was his compassionate acknowledgment that the pain was real and that I was not crazy.

As he does in this important book, Dr. Schechter immediately demystified the body's pain process and experience for me, and he gave me a workable methodology to heal myself, without any medication, body, mind, and spirit. He helped me to understand why my "personality-type" was contributing to my extreme flair-ups of pain. Within days, I was pain-free, and for years now I have been able to

Testimonials from Actual Patients and Professionals

care for myself and follow a system that allows me to live a great life. I am forever grateful."

Peter Capozzi, Executive Producer
The PBS TV show *Jazzy Vegetarian*

"Dr. Schechter has given me the tools to recognize TMS in my patients and together we have helped patients achieve life changing experiences in chronic pain. His approach is unique, empowering, effective, and wellness oriented. I have seen drastic, positive changes in my TMS patients when they see Dr. Schechter. I strongly recommend this important book."

Tara Pollak, DPT, Physical Therapist

"I am writing to express my thanks for helping me achieve what I had previously given up hope on. As you know, before I saw you I had severe back pain and had experienced frustrating episodes of plantar fasciitis and patellar tendinitis dating back to high school. Now I am completely pain free, and I know that I have been cured for good."

J. H., Patient

"I also just wanted to thank Dr. Schechter again because it is thanks to him giving me the correct diagnosis of TMS that I have been able to work full time again for the first time in 12 years! What a joy... Thank you for your important work, it changes people's lives!"

Lisa E., Patient

"I have known Dr. Schechter for over 15 years. This book is a tremendous synthesis of the neuroscience information as it relates to the TMS syndrome. I encourage all clinicians to read this book and improve your clinical practice."

Gerald Edwards, DC, Chiropractor

THINK AWAY YOUR PAIN

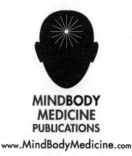

DAVID SCHECHTER, M.D.

MINDBODY
MEDICINE
PUBLICATIONS
www.MindBodyMedicine.com

Think Away Your Pain
Includes bibliographical references.
1. Backache—treatment 2. Chronic Pain-treatment 3. Chronic Pain—psychological aspects. 4. Mind and body 5. Alternative medicine I. Title

ISBN: 978-1-929997-15-2
Library of Congress Control Number: 2014916982

First Printing, 2014
Printed in the United States of America
Interior Design by Gordy Grundy
Cover Design by Gordy Grundy
Photography by Kareem Assassa, The Beverly Hills Photographer
Printed by Bang Printing, Valencia, CA

The information in this book is not offered, nor should it be used by itself to diagnose or treat any particular disease or any particular patient. Neither the author nor the publisher is engaged in rendering professional advice or services to the individual reader. Medical advice should be obtained locally and websites listed in the book and elsewhere provide lists of doctors who can diagnose and treat painful conditions.

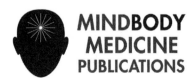

MINDBODY MEDICINE PUBLICATIONS

E-Mail: publisher@MindBodyMedicine.com
10811 Washington Blvd, Suite 250
Culver City, CA 90232
www.MindBodyMedicine.com

DEDICATION

I dedicate this book to my wife **Lisa**. You are my life partner in a voyage that is at times turbulent, often surprising, but always loving.

I also dedicate this book to the thousands of TMS patients who have gone beyond the conventional, been open to change and looked inside themselves. You are far more courageous and special than you even realize.

ACKNOWLEDGMENTS

To John Sarno, M.D., who gave me a special step up in the mind-body healing arena. In 1981, I attended a series of his seminars while a medical student. In 1982, I spent a summer in his office suite, seeing patients and doing research under his direction.

To Gordy Grundy for an amazing job editing and formatting the book. You are a superb book editor and producer, creative and even-tempered.

To Matt Krantz, for the guidance he provided in terms of organization and structure. Matt is the author of *Investing Online for Dummies, Fundamental Analysis for Dummies*, and other books and articles.

To David Shapiro for his amazing edit of the manuscript. Much appreciated. To Janet and Dennis Mendel and Lisa for careful editing of the grammar and word usage. Thanks for your energetic help.

To my growing sons who, in their increasing independence, gave me enough time to finish this book project.

To my office staff, especially Vanessa, for helping me provide the best care that is possible to all of our patients.

To my friend Eric for amusing me a few times a week in phone calls or texts.

To my parents for raising me, muffling their surprise and emphasizing their joy when I became a physician. Those closest to us are our most profound teachers and our most difficult "patients".

ANCIENT AND MODERN
MEDICAL WISDOM

"Study the Patient, rather than the disease."

~ Hippocrates, 450-370 BCE

"... the reason why the cure of many diseases is unknown to the physicians of Hellas, (is) because they are ignorant of the whole, which ought to be studied also; for the part can never be well unless the whole is well."

~ Plato, Charmides, 380 BCE

"The physician should not treat the disease but the patient who is suffering from it."

~ Maimonides (Moses ben Maimon)
Treatise on Asthma, 1190

"The good physician treats the disease, the great physician treats the patient who has the disease."

~ Sir William Osler, 1849-1919

"The doctor may also learn more about the illness from the way the patient tells the story than from the story itself."

~ James B. Herrick, M.D., 1861-1954

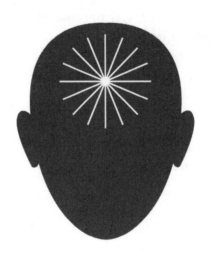

TABLE OF CONTENTS

THINK
AWAY
Y●UR
PAIN

THE SEVEN LESSONS OF PAIN

Lesson One: The source of chronic pain is often the nervous system and brain, not structural injury.

Lesson Two: The context and the interpretation of the pain by the patient and its perceived significance are crucial.

Lesson Three: Psychology and education can change the mind/brain and cure pain, not just manage it.

Lesson Four: Pain does not always mean disease or damage.

Lesson Five: The severity of the pain does not always correlate with the severity of the condition or the potential for damage to the body.

Lesson Six: Pain (sensory) signals are a two-way street. The mind/brain plays a crucial role in what you feel.

Lesson Seven: Mind-body pain keeps coming back until you are firm in your belief that there are no physical causes.

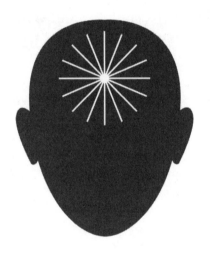

INTRODUCTION

I have written this book because there is in this world:

a) Too much needless suffering from pain.

b) Too many answers, when patients and doctors do not always ask the correct questions.

My goals include:

1) Helping people to find the right approach to relieve their pain.

2) Shifting the dialogue about pain relief to a more natural, more logical, more cost-effective approach for the millions of appropriate sufferers.

3) Countering the effects of our pharmaceutical driven culture, advertising and a medical research climate that ignores or suppresses alternative approaches.

This book addresses the following important concepts in pain diagnosis and treatment:

• Pain is an internationally widespread issue that affects millions of people each year. You are not alone.

• The causes of pain often seem a mystery even as doctors are equipped with advanced imaging technology.

- While doctors often have the best of intentions, they can make pain worse by trying to fix a body that is not really broken.

- The wrong surgery, done for the wrong reasons and failing to correct the problem, can lead to more suffering.

- The mind can create or amplify physical pain. Knowing this may be the solution to your suffering.

- This book can teach you ways to train your mind/brain to be the solution to your pain. (Italicized words are defined in the Glossary at the end of the book.)

If you have picked up this book, chances are that you are currently in pain, frequently suffer from pain, or have a family member or close friend struggling with pain. This is a real and important issue for you. Pain may be destroying your life and you want your life back. I understand what you are feeling because I have talked to and treated thousands of people like you over the past 25 years. The described method has worked for me and so I personally understand its power as well.

Maybe your back hurts so badly you cannot pick up and hug your children. Perhaps it is a stiff neck, a daily headache, or an ache in the jaw. It could be a pain in your pelvis, groin, elbow or chest. Maybe you become nervous every time you need to sneeze, fearing that your back "will go out," and this leads to you having to hobble around for weeks. Some suffer pain so great that even trivial tasks, such as tying shoes, fill them with dread and anxiety. Others give up activities they love, forsaking an active life, fearing that their bodies cannot handle it.

Almost certainly you have seen one, two, or even many doctors for this problem. Probably you have seen alternative practitioners as well, perhaps tried acupuncture and had chiropractic adjustments. You are not alone. Back pain itself is one of the most frequent reasons for visits to the doctor. Other kinds of painful symptoms such as neck pain, tension headaches, arm pain, TMJ jaw pain and more are also extremely common.

If you are picking up this book, it is likely that your medical and surgical doctors have not had an answer. You have probably tried a number of approaches without real success. You may find temporary relief perhaps, but no real sense of getting your life back or gaining control over your pain.

Unfortunately, despite the amazing advances in modern medicine ranging from wiping out smallpox, preventing polio and even allowing the deaf to partially hear, most doctors seem puzzled or limited in their ability to understand and relieve pain without strong painkillers or invasive surgery. If you are like most people, a visit to the doctor for your pain has resulted in a prescription for anti-inflammatory medication or even painkillers, and perhaps an ominous warning to "take it easy." You may have been handed a sheet of paper with some stretches to do at home or referred to physical therapy. And that is if you are lucky.

There is an answer for your pain. I believe many of you will learn that answer in this book and be able to redirect your treatment from what you will learn.

~ David Schechter, M.D.

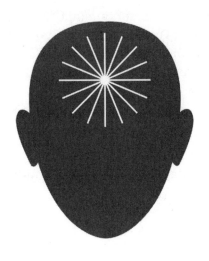

CHAPTER I

Treatments For Pain

There is a lot of research on the treatment of back and neck pain. Yet among consensus recommendations for *acute* (recent) back and neck pain, the best treatment is often little or no treatment. Studies by Daniel Cherkin, Ph.D. and Richard Deyo, M.D., M.P.H., have shown minimal to no difference between chiropractic, medication, or physical therapy for acute pain as compared to a simple educational booklet. (1) (2) (The first use of important or confusing words is italicized and defined in the Glossary.)

Antii Malmivaara, M.D., Ph.D., and his associates in Finland compared bed rest for two days to back exercises and continuation of ordinary activities as tolerated. Those who continued their ordinary activities did the best. (3)

Steven Linton, Ph.D. and his associates in Sweden described in a research paper that early activation reduced the risk of developing chronic pain to 1/8th of usual levels. Movement, not rest, was the answer. (4)

Of course you want to avoid surgery for most chronic pain. Surgery for chronic pain in which parts of your back are "repaired" all too often can lead to a failure to relieve pain and in many cases, make it even worse. Much worse.

This book is not just about back pain. This work is about many types of bodily pain with a focus on *chronic* pain, which can be defined as pain that persists for more than six months. In addition,

1

many of the principles discussed here are quite applicable to pain that lasts an hour, a week or a month.

What Kinds of Pain Are Addressed in This Book?

- Back, neck, buttocks, hip, shoulder pain

- Jaw pain (TMJ)

- Tension headaches and migraines

- Unexplained pelvic pain (women and men)

- Arm pain, "overuse syndromes", tendonitis, Repetitive Strain Injury

- Fibromyalgia pains (a soft tissue pain syndrome)

- Myofascial pain (another kind of soft tissue pain)

- Abdominal pain in children and Irritable Bowel Syndrome pain

- Pain that is not explained

- Pain that is explained but not relieved

THE FAILINGS OF MODERN MEDICINE

Modern medicine has a predisposition to use technology to examine and analyze the body, identify anything that seems wrong, and fix it. As you will learn in this book, the trouble with this approach is not all causes of pain can be seen on an x-ray, MRI, or CT scan of your spine, your arm, or even your abdomen. Also, not everything seen on an x-ray or MRI has any relevance at all to why that individual is in pain. Your body is an incredibly complicated structure that is controlled by the brain and the central nervous system. In brief, the *mind/brain (italicized words defined in Glossary)* exerts its control over the body in ways neither scientists nor most doctors fully understand or have learned to utilize successfully. And many times, it is the mind/brain, not the body, that is responsible for the pain you are suffering from now.

It is precisely in this interplay between the mind and body, the area where our understanding of physiology is the murkiest, that pain and our reaction to it exist. Clinical evidence, brain imaging evidence and other research have been building a powerful case that pain can be understood and can be conquered. (See Chapter VI for discussion of the scientific evidence.)

Often, pain can be solved not with scalpels, pills, or even computers, but by understanding why the brain is continuing to tell us that we hurt, and using this information to consciously send out new information to the nervous system. I call this re-programming your nervous system. A person can learn to do this, and although it is not easy, the practice is natural and successful. When it works, the bodily pain diminishes and often goes away completely.

Unfortunately, medical care often leads first to the pill bottle, a needle-tipped syringe, or the scalpel. Costs and fees are high for invasive procedures. Facility fees alone for surgery or epidural injections can run into the many thousands of dollars. Maybe you are fortunate to have good health insurance, but someone is footing the bill! And invasive does not necessarily mean successful. There are no guarantees.

Doctors, frustrated in dealing with chronic pain, continue to fall back on treatments that do not work. Prescriptions for painkillers rose more than 300 percent between 1999 and 2010. (5) Orders for MRIs and CT scans jumped 57% between 1999 and 2009, based upon the analysis of 23,918 doctor visits for spine problems by four researchers from the Harvard Medical School, including John Mafi, M.D. (6) Doctors took these extreme steps even though the best advice after an initial attack of back pain, is typically some ice, ibuprofen or acetaminophen and to resume one's usual activities as tolerated. (1) (Also see Chapter II.) "Despite numerous published clinical guidelines, management of back pain has relied increasingly on guideline discordant care," the study says. In other words, doctors are trying all sorts of things—often the wrong things.

Furthermore, the results are often inadequate pain relief or even additional pain and suffering at a tremendous cost. A study in 1992 showed that back surgery is often unsuccessful at relieving pain. (7)

Interestingly, back surgery is especially unsuccessful when the patient has suffered childhood psychological distress, according to research by Jerome Schofferman, M.D. and his co-researchers from the San Francisco Spine Institute. (7) Patients who had back surgery reported the results to be unsatisfactory 85% of the time when they had, earlier in their lives, experienced at least three out of five negative experiences. These negative experiences include sexual or physical abuse or other mental trauma. This study suggests that pain continues, even after surgery, when a patient's mind/brain is "in pain." There is no evidence these patients were any different structurally than the successful patients. Surgeons operate on the back, not the mind/brain.

This research suggests that dealing with the negative feelings experienced by a patient could be just as important to the success of a procedure as the technical skill of the surgeon. Other studies have emphasized that surgical outcomes and non-surgical outcomes are about the same after one or two years. (8)

THE NERVOUS SYSTEM. THE MIND.
THE BRAIN. THE EMOTIONS.

Despite the evidence detailed above, doctors, in many cases, are so focused on MRIs of the body and pinpointing physical problems that they are overlooking the real source of the pain. And that is what this book will help you see. Your negative emotions, such as fear, anxiety, stress, grief, anger and panic, trigger real changes in your brain. Your mind/brain sets into motion changes in the mind-body linkage that cause nerves to send pain signals or to amplify existing sensations inappropriately.

I refer to this phenomenon as TMS. I use the acronym to credit John Sarno, M.D., for his pioneering discoveries in this field. His analyses are such that if fully appreciated they would merit a Nobel Prize for Medicine or similar award.

I will discuss the description and explanation for pain that he called Tension Myositis (or Myoneural) Syndrome (TMS). Others have used this terminology and have also used other names including Distraction Pain Syndrome (DPS) (9), Psychophysiological Pain Disorder (PPD) (10), and The Mindbody Syndrome. For many of these phrases, the TMS acronym works well. But whatever we call it, or however you have heard it described, the most important fact is that your brain might very well be why you are in pain.

For over twenty-five years, I have been successfully treating and teaching patients to end their pain. This book will teach you how to do it. As a result of many years of research, this book brings together many ideas and concepts that I have used to successfully treat patients. My goal here is to begin with the groundbreaking work of Dr. John Sarno and break some further ground in the search for the truth in the cause and treatment of chronic pain.

I have now treated well over two thousand patients in my practice with this methodology. My patients have a high success rate of improving and a remarkable rate of cure. (11) My methods have evolved somewhat over the years, but the basic principles remain similar. Diagnosis and treatment are fundamentally a medical process and yet both have a remarkably different focus than that which is familiar to you. Tens of thousands more have been helped by my prior works *The MindBody Workbook, The MindBody Audio Program,* and *The MindBody Patient Panel.* (12, 13, 14) I am writing this book to synthesize what I have learned over these years and put it in a useful, understandable and workable form for you to read, study and practice. *Think Away Your Pain* represents my up-to-date knowledge, techniques and understanding to treat pain by focusing on the mind, brain and emotions.

HOW THE MIND CAUSES PAIN:
A DRAMATIC EXAMPLE

All this might sound great in theory, but you may still have lingering doubts. I have had great success helping patients conquer chronic back pain and a myriad of other painful conditions by helping them understand the mental connection, rather than rely on purely physical treatments. A great TMS success is one in which a patient is diagnosed with this condition after many years of suffering unnecessarily and the result is the elimination of pain and disability. My perspective differs from that of many doctors. I find that the patient who has failed many treatments, but is open to this one, presents a high likelihood of success, rather than a likely failure. That is because failing at other approaches, and therefore feeling desperate, may make this individual the ideal patient for this diagnosis and treatment.

A powerful story of what is wrong with the way modern medicine deals with pain is evident in the example of a woman who came to my office a year or two ago. (The details of all the cases in this book have been changed for anonymity and may represent composites of one or more patients for illustration purposes.) She was a professional woman, about 45 years old, well-dressed, successful and articulate, except that she had one problem: crippling back pain. This patient was intrigued about what she had heard of the work I do trying to understand how the mind/brain can actually create (and therefore cure) physical pain. She came to me for help.

Accompanied by her adult daughter, this patient told my assistant her rather lengthy history, after which I began my own discussion with her. Notably, she recalled excruciating *sciatica* (leg pain shooting from the back or buttocks) starting the day after she received horrible, traumatic personal news. The day before this crippling pain flared up, she found out that her ex-husband had died suddenly and tragically.

The death occurred some seven or so years before she saw me and her physical pain began the day after she received the news of her ex-husband. A friend even commented to her that it must be due to the traumatic news, but at that point she was unable to process that connection. How could such severe pain be caused by her own mind?

The initial pain continued for several weeks and then she saw a spine surgeon with whom she was acquainted socially. He examined her and obtained an MRI, which showed, reportedly, a small disc bulge. She pleaded with him to relieve her pain, now torturing her for nearly four weeks. At this time, only some medication had been tried. No other conservative therapy of any kind was attempted. The psychological trauma was not explored at all.

The spine surgeon advised surgery and this was done about a month after the onset of the pain, a month and one day after the news of her spouse's death. Of course, studies have shown that bulges in discs do not necessarily translate into an explanation for a patient's pain. (See Chapter VI.) Not surprisingly, the surgery was ineffective and did not relieve her leg pain.

The pain persevered and her search for a solution continued. Her journey consisted of visits to a half-dozen spine doctors, mostly surgeons, in at least two states. This successful businesswoman was respected in her community and very articulate. I am sure her pleadings for pain relief evoked a strong desire to help on the part of her physicians. Nonetheless, not one had obtained a detailed psychosocial history at any point.

She saw one spine surgeon in another state who performed a number of tests including a *discogram*, where dye is injected into one or more of the spinal disks, and concluded that she should *not* have surgery. She continued to search for an answer that led her to another ineffective surgery and six epidural injections, which brought brief but no lasting relief.

Finally, she met with a surgeon at a prominent medical center in Southern California. The surgeon said he was fairly confident that her problem was due to a cyst in her back, adjacent to a nerve, and that surgery could fix her pain. She prepared for her third spinal surgery.

After the operation, the surgeon came back to talk to her, surrounded by several fellows and residents. He confessed that he had cut through a portion of her nerve and that she would have pain in her foot for the rest of her life. In trying to fix her leg and back pain, she wound up adding foot pain to the list. The patient was of course disheartened, but again, forgiving of the surgeon's error. She had been able to forgive everyone involved in her case.

INVESTIGATING HOW THE MIND
CAN HURT THE BODY

When this patient came to me, she was desperately open to another approach. Soon, she began to realize that she needed to get to the root of the problem, not her back, but her mind.

I started with a history and a physical examination. We talked a little more about her life, her concerns and her successes. I reviewed her previous MRI reports and CD images and I performed a detailed physical examination. She was able to touch the floor and had good back extension as well. Three surgeries had inactivated her Achilles reflex on the right side and she did have hypersensitivity of the right outside (lateral) foot. Otherwise she had a normal neurological exam. She looked younger and more fit than her stated age.

Whenever I suspect the mind is at the root of the pain, I examine what are called *TMS tender points*. These are six areas of the neck, mid back and gluteal muscle, (three on each side) which are often sore to the touch in a pain patient when the mind/brain is the actual cause. (See illustration Chapter VIII.) TMS causes the mind to constrict blood flow to various parts of the back (not just the painful ones) resulting in tenderness. It is something a trained physician can quickly detect. With this patient, her TMS tender points were quite evident in four of the classically described six spots.

More important than anything I found with the woman's body is what she said during the exam. During the medical interview in my office, this patient shared a revelation. She noted her former spouse had tried to get back together with her several times, but they remained good friends. She resisted getting back together because of his personal issues and demons. He was an alcoholic and exhibited erratic behavior as a result. My patient felt guilty that her former spouse's death might have been her fault. She worried that she did not do enough for him. Notably, her grown daughter, sitting beside her, did not blame her mother for her father's death in any way. Thus, potent and self-destructive guilt was the patient's real problem, not her body.

TEACHING THE MIND TO HEAL THE BODY

Do you see a bit of yourself in this patient? Her story is a classic example of intense concern for others and a tendency to be hard on oneself, called *goodism*. *Goodism* is a key trait that triggers TMS and was readily apparent in this case. It is just one personality trait that tends to appear in people who suffer from TMS, as you will find out about later in this book. (See Chapter VIII.)

Bottled up inside this woman was agonizing guilt. She was quite willing to forgive everyone, even the doctors who steered her wrong and compounded her pain. She forgave everyone except the most important person in her life: Herself. Her inability to forgive herself, to ease off her own self-criticism and guilt, was an ongoing feature of her predicament.

Rather than seeking more surgery, this patient sought to understand how her mind was causing the pain. Now that this patient understood that it was not her body causing the pain, she set about finding a solution inside her mind. Some of the things she did are treatment methods that I describe later in this book. (See Chapter X.) The most important realization in the healing process is recognizing that your mind can both hurt you and it can cure you. This was certainly the case here.

After my diagnosis, the patient followed up with me a month after she started her TMS treatment. She happily reported that she was feeling better than she had in quite a while. She still struggled to convince herself that mental worry and stress could cause back pain, but the fact that she was already getting better was starting to win her over.

How did she conquer her pain? She followed the steps that you can learn in this book. Among these steps include:

• Find out more about TMS. I often have my patients read one of the books written by Dr. John Sarno and will now have them read this book as well. As the pioneer in this field, Sarno's insights are valuable and his perspective unique. Other home study materials are advised, including an audio program and DVD, which I created for home use. (13)

• Write in a journal. You may have kept a diary when you were young, but might not have seen how writing down your feelings can have a healing power. The problem is many of us are too busy to sit down and start writing or typing our feelings on a blank sheet of paper. A guided set of self-assessment questions is the core of my *MindBody Workbook* (14), which is designed to get people thinking about their emotions, not their pain. The workbook asks questions to help you get to the core of emotional issues or triggers that puts TMS into motion.

• Study the "Twelve Stages of Healing." There are twelve steps that TMS sufferers often pass on the journey to conquer their pain. When dealing with the mind, it is natural to encounter various challenges in healing. These include the ups and downs and even doubting the diagnosis, both of which commonly face the recovering pain patient. (See Chapter X.)

• Seek therapy. No, not physical therapy but mental therapy. No amount of stretching, breathing or sun salutations were going to take away the guilt of her ex-spouse's untimely end. The patient found a therapist, on her own, who was trying to work within this model. There are also specialized therapists who understand how the mind can create pain. (See Chapter XIII.)

This patient left my office optimistic, as was I, that the path I had guided her to would be a successful one. She understood that there was work to do in order to undo the negative effects of the past and to create a positive future.

This story illustrates how pain is not necessarily caused by a gnarled spine or a bulged disc. In fact, those issues are rare and not the key cause of pain. It turns out that some people are programmed with personality traits that make it more likely that their mind will cause them pain.

WHAT DOES ALL THIS MEAN FOR ME?

How can the world's most advanced medical community make such a massive mistake? Why are we spending billions on procedures that do not take away pain, and in many cases, make it worse? The answer is that doctors are trained to look for problems in the body as the causes of pain. But when the mind, the brain and the emotions are the root cause, it is usually missed.

Through years of working with patients and teaching them to help themselves, I have created a roadmap for healing. It is not a pill you can ingest or an injection you receive. It is a regimen that requires you to dive into your mind, understand what pains you emotionally, and examine the features of your personality that make you a candidate for TMS. It is unlikely that you have ever embarked upon such a process after visiting with a doctor. And that is because to cure your body, you have to cure your mind. You can learn to *THINK AWAY YOUR PAIN*.

THINK DIFFERENTLY ABOUT YOUR PAIN

Most pain psychologists take as a given that a patient's pain cannot be fixed by psychological methods and approaches. Their goal is to teach behavioral techniques to manage, control and adapt to the pain.

This is where I differ. I do believe psychology can cure pain. That is just one of the things I have discovered about pain, which I have highlighted as the Seven Lessons of Pain. You will find out about all seven in this book, but for now, I'd like you to think about Lesson Three. Lesson Three is the key to unlocking your ability to let this book help you. In Lesson Three, you will learn that psychology and education can cure pain, not just manage it.

Lesson Three: Psychology and education can change the mind/brain and cure pain, not just manage it.

HOW THIS BOOK WILL GUIDE YOU

Think of this book as your map to begin healing your pain.

This book begins by explaining the basics of pain. The more you learn about this the better. I will teach it to you in a way that you can understand your pain in an up-to-date and important way.

You will also understand what rare physical conditions can legitimately trigger physical pain and why surgery in those very unusual cases might be needed.

Next, the book dives into the mental aspect of pain. You will see how modern medicine has been unlocking the evidence some doctors have suspected all along, that your mind and emotions can make you hurt.

Once you have understood what causes pain and how the mind is in control, it is time to create a detailed plan of attack to banish it. The next section of the book dives into the Twelve Stages of Healing in full detail. Each step will give you a specific message that I use with patients to reduce or eliminate their pain.

This book looks into the future by showing how research continues to unlock secrets of the mind and its connection to pain. I even have a section whose focus is on doctors and health care practitioners who want to learn more about this. It may also be of interest to the general reader for whom this book is intended.

Inspirational quotes and stories from patients who have succeeded also appear near the end of the book. I believe these can inspire you to do the work required to succeed and may inspire other doctors to take the plunge with their patients as well.

HOW TO READ THIS BOOK FOR THE MOST BENEFIT

There are different ways to read this book:

1) Some may wish to read straight through the book.

2) Others may wish to begin with Patient Stories (Chapter VII) and proceed to the Twelve Stages of Healing. (Chapter X)

3) Scientifically minded individuals and health care professionals may find Chapter VI (Evidence), Chapter XI (Research) and Chapter XII (Helping Doctors Learn) most important.

4) Or you can find your own way through the material, take your time and reflect on what you have read.

Careful review and reflection will allow the new and powerful ideas to penetrate profoundly. This deep learning will be the transforming agent in changing your mind/brain, and in doing so, relieve your pain.

Reading this book is a major part of the healing process and here are some other suggestions:

(a) If you read something and think to yourself, "I already know that," do not skip over or dismiss it. Your path to being pain-free involves relearning what you already know and replacing old beliefs with new understandings.

(b) Do not give up just because a week or two has gone by and you are not thinking or feeling differently. The process of healing is a long journey, longer for some than others. Some people experience transformation in a day, in a week, and for some, it may take months. Think about how long it has taken to develop the conditions that now manifest as your pain. It may not take long to heal the pain, but there is some real effort involved in changing your thinking at a deep level. **Be patient, and stick with it!**

(c) Try to find yourself in the book's anecdotal examples. Do you notice some common personality traits? Do you see a similar childhood history? Are you likely to handle stress in a similar way?

Finally, I want you to approach your problem of pain with hope. I have seen this method work for many thousands of people. The first step is to embark on this journey with determination, diligence and openness. You will find insights and great benefit. So let us get started on this healing journey right now!

CHAPTER II

What is Pain?

Understanding Acute and Chronic Pain and the Transition Between the Two

Pain can be debilitating. If you twist your ankle or knee or suffer something more serious, the initial reaction can be to panic. The tendency to fret over pain is especially common when you lose your mobility. But while fear may be your initial reaction, it is not the best one. And if you are in pain, it is best to approach the discomfort in a logical and informed way. In this chapter, you will understand why you get attacked with short-term pain and how it can lead to a long-term affliction. More importantly, you will learn:

• Pain is a normal function of the body. This understanding will help you end your panic over the acute attack.

• Pain is more complex than commonly believed. You will learn why this is actually a key to conquering it.

• Doctors often have the best of intentions. By trying to fix a body that is not really broken, they can make the pain worse.

• Pain usually goes away. The transition from acute pain to chronic pain—*Chronification*—is a key concept in understanding pain.

• The mind can create or amplify physical pain. Once you

understand this, it can be the solution to your suffering!

• This book can help you learn to train your brain to think away the pain.

If you are like most people, pain is not something that is front and center until you have suffered from it. Nearly all of us have suffered a temporary, or *acute*, episode of pain. *(See Glossary, if desired. First use of every glossary word is italicized.)* When you were younger, you probably had your share of scrapes and bumps, but never really worried about them for long because a kiss from your mother, a small bandage and a promise that the pain would go away were all you needed to put your worries to rest.

As we get older, acute attacks can become more severe due to de-conditioning and longer healing times. For many of us, the agony is much scarier because we worry that this is the time the pain will not go away. Be it "throwing out your back," suffering from a tennis elbow flare-up or headache, the acute episode can be agonizing. If the pain is in our chest, that brings up a whole different set of concerns, especially for men over forty. We worry about a heart attack and wonder if we should seek immediate help. Thinking the worst is called *catastrophizing*, a very important concept.

COSTS OF PAIN TO YOU

You may have noticed from first-hand experience, friends or the media that *chronic* pain is a perplexing, disturbing and life-altering condition. Pain can cost you your job, produce huge medical bills, strain your marriage or even lead to depression.

When an attack is unexpected and therefore frightening, many patients head down the long road of lasting pain, even though the pain should pass quickly. For most individuals, the pain is caused by a muscle spasm. The muscle tightens up, clenches and hurts. The good news is that it will go away. The bad news is it may hurt quite a bit until it does.

I do not mean to belittle the acute attack. During an acute attack, you might experience pain that takes your breath away. Some patients with low back pain report crawling, in agony, on their hands and knees to the bathroom. Others are in so much pain they cannot get into bed; they wind up tossing and turning all night on the floor. Others with elbow pain might have difficulty writing, making a phone call or texting. Neck pain can totally eliminate your ability to turn your neck or sleep comfortably.

How you react during those first few critical hours, days and weeks after an acute attack is extremely important. Understanding an acute attack is part of the healing process, even if your pain has not gone away and you are still in a negative pain feedback loop.

You are not a coward because you hate the pain you have experienced. Back spasms, for example, are among the most painful agonies a human can experience. Back pain is right up there with compound fractures, childbirth, passing a kidney stone and cancer pain. Try to keep a perspective that many of these painful events, such as childbirth or a kidney stone, are temporary and do not typically cause long-term damage. Except in the case of some cancers, all these pains come and go. And in most cases, after the acute attack, the patient is none the worse and, in some cases, better. For example, after the distress of childbirth, a baby is born and a woman becomes a loving mother. After passing a kidney stone, a man is greatly relieved, alas without a cute souvenir of this painful, but typically not damaging, episode.

Lesson Four: Pain does not always mean disease or damage.

Back spasms can cause terrible pain as muscles scream out for oxygen, plead for a massage, demand some ice, ibuprofen or anything that will bring relief. Again, in a few hours, days or weeks at most, people are moving around easily. Most tension headaches, pelvic pains and tendonitis have the same pattern. This book deals mostly with long-term, **chronic** or recurring pain, which is, in a sense, an acute attack gone bad.

The process of beating pain starts with how you deal with acute attacks. Maybe you are suffering from one now. The acute attack can be frightening and debilitating. The point of this section is to help you stop the acute attack from turning into a long-term problem. If you are already in long-term pain, I will show you how that very first attack might have been all it took for your brain and nervous system to create a bigger problem.

PAIN IS A SIGNAL

Even if you have been in pain for years, if you are like most people, you can usually trace your pain to a single incident or period of time in your life. Some people tell me that they felt a sudden and distinct pop in their back or neck, which triggered a pain they had never experienced before. Some report hearing a snapping sound or feeling a dull ache that intensified for days following a particularly rousing round of golf. You might also recall a certain summer when you were especially active with sports and wound up with a sore elbow or neck, not to mention a nasty sunburn.

Most long-term pain has to start somewhere and that somewhere is the acute attack. The acute attack is the initial episode of pain that often seems to begin with a specific physical event. It does not have to be the result of high-intensity exercise, such as scaling Mount Everest or running a marathon. Sometimes, frustratingly, an acute attack can be the result of something as simple as picking up a bag of groceries or squeezing a telephone between your shoulder and ear for too long.

Knowing what causes the pain that you are feeling will help you understand how to react to it. Acute pain is due to nerve endings that are sending very intense signals to alert the brain to respond. This does not mean severe damage is occurring.

Pain is a signal. In the short term, its function is to compel you to act in one way. If the pain continues, the signaling gets more complicated and something structurally significant does need to be excluded. But often when the pain persists, the message is more subtle and psychological.

Human beings need pain as a *sensory stimulus* to help avoid danger and respond to injury. One example that illustrates this value is an individual who touches a hot pot on the stove or gets too close to a flame. The body is hardwired to recoil from danger, preventing serious damage. The short-term, intense, acute pain is worth the price as it avoids bigger problems.

Immediately, even prior to the awareness of the pain, a reflex arc of sensory and motor nerves sends signals from the hand to the spinal cord and back which trigger a withdrawal response to avoid further injury. We learn to avoid overly hot objects by experiencing this pain.

INABILITY TO SENSE PAIN

Pain sensation is very important. People can die when pain signaling does not function correctly. While you are suffering from too much pain, believe it or not, there are some people who suffer from not experiencing enough pain!

A common example of this is *diabetic neuropathy*, a serious complication experienced by some diabetes sufferers. After many years of living with the disease, diabetics often develop damage to nerves called neuropathy. As a result of this damage, the nerves lose the ability to send signals to the brain about sensation. Eventually even pain fibers are lost. This means that these people are not able to feel pain or even a light touch to the affected areas.

Thus, a diabetic can get burned more easily on the feet where this condition is most commonly found and is prone to severe burns as a result. Diabetics can also get scratches and puncture wounds that lead to infections on their feet that can progress to *osteomyelitis*, or bone infection, and may require amputations, cause blood poisoning and even death. Therefore, not being able to feel acute pain can have severe side effects.

A small number of people are born without the ability to feel pain properly or even at all. Perhaps 80-100 individuals in the United States have *congenital insensitivity to pain with anhidrosis*, referred to as CIPA. (1) In another and perhaps related condition called *dysautonomia*, a child's ability to feel pain is limited and distorted.

For these unfortunate individuals, many ordinary activities pose a danger of burns, cuts, blood loss, infection or death. Research on this uncommon group of sufferers can help scientists to understand the basic mechanisms of pain. This can be useful for the rest of us.

THE CATEGORIES OF PAIN

When you go to the doctor with the sniffles (nasal congestion), there's no mystery about what the problem is. You most likely either have a viral or mild bacterial infection that simply needs to run its course. A lot of testing is hardly worth the time, except in severe cases, because doctors know what's going on and there's often not much they can do to help anyway. Or the treatment is worse than the disease (e.g. resistant organisms from too many antibiotics).

Unfortunately physical pain isn't so cut-and-dried. Lots of things can hurt and sometimes in more than one area at a time.

Doctors categorize pain into one of three categories, defined by how long it lasts:

• Acute Pain. Pain that lasts for less than a few weeks or up to six weeks is usually defined as acute pain. Acute pain typically comes from trauma, falls, burns, injuries, twists and sprains... and sometimes TMS.

• Sub-Acute Pain. Pain that lasts more than six weeks and up to three months (some say six months) is called sub-acute. This category includes those annoying pulled hamstrings that don't heal, more severe burns that ache, some fractures that mend slowly, some whiplashes that are sore and stiff longer (Myofascial pain) and sometimes TMS.

• Chronic Pain. Once the pain has persisted more than three months (or six months by some definitions) we are dealing with a whole new condition called chronic pain. Chronic pain can last for years or rarely for a lifetime. But in many cases, it need not last at all. In my experience, there is a higher chance statistically this is TMS.

UNDERSTANDING THE ACUTE ATTACK

Pain is the body's way of getting your attention. And it is highly effective, to which most of you can readily attest. Abdominal pain from an early appendicitis can alert us to go to the doctor, have an examination and, if necessary, an operation to treat this condition before it worsens. Should the appendix rupture, the risk of serious illness or even dying is much greater and the treatment required to survive is far more complex.

More subtle joint pain can alert us to the fact that our joints are not as young or supple as they once were. This leads us to logical approaches, such as stretching before sports, running on softer surfaces, getting better shoes or orthotics, and strengthening the muscles to reduce the stress on our joints.

Even when we strain our backs, that pain, as agonizing as it might be, is your body's self-protection mechanism. If you did overextend and cause a microscopic tear in a muscle, the intense pain is designed to get you to stop what you were doing. The subsequent swelling after a knee injury is highly effective in immobilizing you. Your body wants you to stop doing what you were doing to prevent further injury. If someone tells you to "take it easy," you can ignore that. But you cannot easily ignore the searing pain in your muscles.

What we can learn from these examples is that while pain certainly hurts, it is also very important to the long-term protection of your body. The capacity to feel pain is a part of our nervous system that can have a protective role when it is working normally. When you pull a muscle, you listen to your body and let the muscle repair itself. It almost always does.

COMMON REACTIONS TO PAIN ATTACKS

Why is back pain, caused by a sudden spasm of muscles, so frightening? For one thing, the pain is literally behind you. If it is pelvic pain, it is beneath you. If it is chest pain, it implies a heart attack. If it is a headache, well, we're all pretty sensitive about that part of our body too. Back pain is something that you cannot see, but feel and this is part of why it can be scary. Making things worse, you do not know what the pain is telling you or how long it will last. Misinformation only fuels the fear, as you have probably heard horror stories about people with really long term pain problems. You may even worry that the acute attack may represent the first step toward that kind of chronic pain or incapacity. We fear ending up permanently in a wheelchair. Don't worry; back spasms or a herniated disc will not put you there.

Another problem with a "back attack" is that it can happen again. Your doctor might have even scared you, saying something like "Once it happens, it is likely to happen again." It is true that acute attacks can reoccur, but typically with the same result: resolution and return to normal activity. Fear, avoidance of activity and poor treatment, can lead to more episodes or even worse, chronic pain. (2)

If you have had not one or two but a few of these attacks and you do not understand the mind-body connection, you may start to baby your back, calf or hip. You may avoid activity, telling people that you have a bad back, and, in so doing, you might be unknowingly setting yourself up for more problems. Most of this pain is muscular, in the soft tissue, and it goes away. Being more flexible, physically and emotionally, can help. Sitting less and being more physically active can make a difference as well.

I see people in the office who move like a stiff robot when I ask them to bend over. They control every centimeter of movement and typically limit themselves far before they reach their usual flexibility limits. With a diagnosis of TMS and appropriate treatment, I typically observe that they move more fluidly at each subsequent visit. This parallels their clinical improvement and increased emotional confidence. Some of these folks have been *guarding* or moving very restrictedly for years before I first examine them. And it all starts with a single event, a pain attack of one kind or another in which they have experienced severe or excruciating back pain, sometimes radiating to the buttocks, thighs or lower legs.

WHAT TO DO WHEN ACUTE PAIN STRIKES

This is not a book about dealing with sprains and strains. There is plenty of advice on the Internet or from your doctor. If your pain is just an acute, self-limited attack and you look at it this way, you would never really need to read this book.

Acute pain is part of being human. In fact, the amount of time a person has been in pain is a big factor in how I initially diagnose and treat it. Acute pain is kind of like the common cold. There is not much doctors really need to advise, other than recommend the tried-and-true message of RICE: Relative Rest, Ice, Compression and Elevation. For most people, time and RICE will solve the pain. To the "R," I would add Reassurance, the guiding touch that helps a patient to understand that the pain is going to end and one is going to recover completely. You would be amazed at the effectiveness of a doctor's kind words; acute pain will go away and recovery time is lessened.

Still, some doctors love to prescribe rest, even though this has proven to be the wrong approach in most cases. (3) After all, that is the "R" in RICE. Patients usually love to be prescribed rest. The best way to speed recovery after suffering an acute attack of *benign* pain, not of a serious cause, is to keep rest to a relative minimum. You must try to get back to what you were doing before, as fast as you are able to. Too much rest can reinforce a pain cycle. Our mind/brain begins to think of itself as "injured" or "damaged" and this becomes a self-perpetuating cycle that can lead to mind-body dysfunction.

Reduce your level of activity a little. Resume usual activities as soon as you are able. Ice and anti-inflammatory medications like ibuprofen and naproxen (Advil and Aleve) are a reasonable, short-term approach to bring the pain down to a manageable, tolerable level while the painful area heals. And it almost always does.

Now, if you are sure it is a TMS flare-up, there is even a better way to deal with this, with the mind. More will follow on this later.

WHEN PAIN BECOMES CHRONIC:
INTRODUCTION TO CHRONIFICATION

It is in those rarer cases when the pain does not go away, that the *mind/brain* starts to get involved. This is called the *chronification* of pain. And that is exactly what we are trying to avoid.

Chronification is a funny sounding and somewhat awkward word that describes an important process. The process is the transition from acute or sub-acute pain into chronic pain. The transition begins when the patient and his doctor believe the pain is going away and evolves into something else, where doubt has crept in and the condition just does not seem to want to heal.

It would be great if there were a vaccine against this, wouldn't it? There is an alternative. It is knowledge, understanding and reassurance, at the proper time, by the proper person or book, in the proper way. It also helps if the patient is receptive to this message. Sometimes when we are overwhelmed, stressed, burned out or frustrated, we may not be in the right place to hear this message, no matter how well stated.

With an acute attack of back pain, the affliction may typically last from a few days up to six weeks, without special knowledge or treatment. As mentioned previously, most of these pains resolve, regardless of treatment. Less is often more.

Things get complicated when a patient's acute pain does not go away. The patient's mind starts racing. "Will I walk normally again?" "Will I ever be able to play sports?" "Will I be able to pick up my grandkids?" These questions of doubt and worry flood the mind. And before long, some patients are literally transforming unconsciously. This is catastrophizing. Thinking the worse about the pain. What could have been a brief attack transitions into something more. Enter chronic pain.

Once patients start worrying and fearing the effects of that initial attack, the pain is at more risk of turning into something else. We have learned from the Northwestern researchers that chronic pain is generated from a different part of the brain than acute pain. Chronic pain comes from the same area of the brain that contains "emotion-related circuitry." (4) Patients with chronic pain have a different problem and therefore need a different solution than people who have an acute injury.

Acute pain can be treated in a variety of ways or often not at all. Individuals heal and get well. One recent study found that infants given sucrose during a painful procedure cried much less than those who did not. (5) Short-term pain can be treated with some TLC. "A spoonful of sugar," usually a tablet of aspirin or a massage, can definitely help one get over the immediate pain from a twisted ankle. However, once pain becomes chronic, it is a different "animal." The focus must be the emotional, *not* just the physical. In fact, we focus away from the structural and on to the psychological in order to get great results in treatment.

CHRONIC PAIN: CATEGORIES AND DEEPER UNDERSTANDING

Let us take a step back and analyze why an individual might suffer from longer lasting or chronic pain. Chronic pain is defined as pain lasting three to six months or more. I think of it as indicative of one of the following three categories or issues:

a) The condition causing the pain has not been effectively treated.

b) The condition cannot be cured.

c) The cause of the pain is more complex than suspected and is rooted in the way the brain and nervous system works.

Let us look at each of these categories one at a time.

PAIN NOT EFFECTIVELY TREATED

An example of this would be an unsuccessful surgery on the gallbladder where a gallstone was left in the common bile duct. The pain persists, despite surgery and becomes chronic. A skilled clinician will determine that the reason for the pain is the persistent stone and the treatment may be a procedure, like an *ERCP* that removes the stone and therefore relieves the pain.

Other examples would be a surgical sponge left inside the body during an operation or a piece of shrapnel, missed when a gunshot wound was explored.

PAIN THAT CANNOT BE CURED

An example of pain that perhaps cannot be cured is the unfortunate circumstance of metastatic cancer. If cancer has spread far from its original source, it may not always be possible to cure the disease. Fortunately, there are more and more examples of success today.

Pain may become chronic as the bony metastases hurt the patient. The pain can be controlled by medications such as morphine or radiation treatment, but the cause cannot be cured. These types of chronic pain have a relatively clear explanation once the doctor does the tests and figures out the cause. Thankfully, cancer as the cause of chronic pain is statistically rare.

PAIN WHOSE CAUSE IS MORE COMPLEX AND BRAIN RELATED

Other types of chronic pain have more complex explanations. Two examples that illustrate both the peculiarity and complexity of pain, while also showing us the importance of the brain and central nervous system in pain, are *Phantom limb pain* and *Referred pain*.

PHANTOM LIMB PAIN

Phantom leg pain is fascinating in helping us to understand chronic pain. When an individual has part of a leg amputated for trauma, diabetes, circulatory problems or other reasons, there is a condition called "phantom limb pain" that can develop.

The "phantom" in "phantom limb pain" refers to the fact that the normal leg is no longer there in its entirety. The pain is felt by the patient as if their leg, or sometimes the ankle or foot, hurts. But there is no ankle or foot on that side. The patient is aware of the lack of the structure but distinctively reports that it hurts. Are they crazy? Abso-

27

lutely not. They are having a real phenomenon that is often chronic called Phantom Limb Pain.

What is phantom limb pain all about? There are a number of theories and explanations for this type of pain. One explanation focuses on the nerve endings at the point at which the leg was cut off. These nerve endings are fully connected to the remainder of the leg and to the sciatic nerve, spinal cord and brain. However, at the site where the amputation occurred, they are cut without connections to other structures. They may even ball up at this end, "stump neuroma." This explanation posits that this jumble of information leads to errant signals that the brain misinterprets as pain. (6)

A more sophisticated explanation requires the understanding of how and where sensory signals are interpreted in the brain. Different parts of the brain detect and analyze the signals from various parts of the body.

As a result of examining patients with different types of brain problems, such as tumors and strokes, doctors have been able to map out the pattern of these signals. In the brain, portions of the sensory cortex correspond to various parts of the body such as our face, hands, feet and much more. The body parts that are densely packed with nerve endings, such as fingertips, lips and tongue, dominate this area in relation to other body parts with less nerve stimulation.

Typically, signals are constantly being sent to the brain. When an amputation occurs, the associated area of the brain stops receiving information, neither normal pain nor dysfunction signals. According to this explanation, the brain eventually goes haywire. It begins to interpret the lack of signals and perhaps confuses a combination of them. Thus, the patient feels "phantom pain." (7)

It is quite important to understand this clearly: the patient had an amputation. It healed well. There is a clean, dry stump. But the patient's "foot" on that side of his body hurts. The persistent pain is NOT from the foot nor a diseased, damaged structure. The pain ultimately is caused by the way the nervous system has a dysfunction and the way the brain incorrectly interprets this information.

The condition is treatable. The stump is carefully examined and if a nerve mass or neuroma has developed, it may be injected or surgically removed to treat the persisting pain. The patient may also be given medication that reduces the sensitivity of nerve sensations at the nerve and brain level. This reduces the experience of pain. Cognitive psychotherapy and patient education can also help the patient to reinterpret these new sensations as something benign and not dangerous. This can further reduce the problem. More recently, mirror therapy has been used to change the sensory signals to the brain by tricking it into seeing the bad leg as the good one (in the mirror). (8) (9)

Phantom leg pain is fascinating in helping us to understand chronic pain. It illustrates two of the several key principles that I am emphasizing in this book:

Lesson Four: Pain does not always mean disease or damage.

Lesson One: The source of chronic pain is often the nervous system and brain, not structural injury.

REFERRED PAIN

Another concept which exemplifies the complexity of the brain and nervous system and their relationship to pain is referred pain. Referred pain means pain that is not felt at the location of the problem but is instead felt somewhere else along a related nerve tract.

Heart attack pain can hurt in the left arm or up to the neck and jaw. This can be in addition to chest pressure. The reason for this referred pain is that the sensory fibers, which provide nerve contact with the heart muscle, are branches of nerves, which go to the arm, neck and jaw. The latter branches get much more activation than the heart branches do, because our arm, neck and jaw send many signals to the brain in relationship to our daily activities like eating and moving.

Fortunately, we are much less aware of our heart muscle. When a heart attack occurs, the heart muscle has insufficient oxygen and is threatened with cellular death. The sensations that are sent from the heart are sometimes interpreted as related to the arm, neck and jaw. Occasionally we feel nausea and shortness of breath as well. If someone is not aware of these atypical symptoms, they may delay care that is urgently needed. The teaching point here is that:

The location of the problem does not always match the location of the pain.

Another related issue is the intensity of the pain. Some patients with a heart attack, at least initially, describe relatively mild sensations. The potential for severe damage to the heart muscle, or even death, is quite high. On the other hand, the severe pain of re-nal colic (kidney stones,) is described by many as 10 out of 10 on a pain scale. This is perhaps equivalent to the intense sensation of childbirth. In these latter examples of childbirth and kidney stones, the potential for damage to the body is much lower than the pain intensity indicates.

Another example is back spasms. These can be excruciating and can force a grown man down on his knees in seconds. I have had patients unable to rise from the floor to get to a bed or chair, even for hours after being hit with back spasms. Typically, in a few days the patient is better and it is not unusual for them to be completely normal, pain free and active in a few short weeks!

On the other hand, a patient with a more severe spinal con-dition, such as spinal stenosis, may have subtle numbness in a big toe or a mild visual disturbance as the initial manifestation. These examples support this important lesson:

Lesson Five: The severity of the pain does not always correlate with the severity of the condition or the potential for damage to the body.

We have learned that:

a) Pain does not always mean disease.

b) The mind can sometimes be the source of pain.

c) The location of the pain does not always match the location of a physical problem.

d) The severity of the pain does not always correlate with the severity of a physical condition or the potential for physical damage.

To better understand points C and D, we need to recognize that the context of an injury plays an enormous role in how one experiences pain.

THE EXPERIENCE OF PAIN: THE CONTEXT IS CRUCIAL

You are about to read two stories of identical men who experienced similar injuries in very different circumstances. As you are reading them, look for how the change in the context of the injury has a huge effect on the experience of pain.

Story One: A Traumatic Injury with Minimal Pain

A 19-year-old young man, Sean, has just spent three months on patrols in Afghanistan. Rooting out terrorists and avoiding roadside bombs is difficult and stressful work. Sean has begun to question whether he is in the right career. He is burned out on the long days, tense nights and the experience of witnessing his buddies fall with injuries or worse. Unexpectedly, while his squad is on routine patrol, an enemy sniper fires at them. Sean feels a burning pain as a bullet hits his foot, probably breaking a toe or metatarsal (a foot bone).

Surprisingly, having survived the encounter, the soldier is feeling quite calm and the pain is tolerable. The medic attends to the bleeding by removing his shoe and bandaging the wound. The injured soldier is taken back to base in a Humvee, cared for by a corpsman and a doctor. It is determined that he will need foot surgery. A helicopter is summoned to take him to Bagram Air Force base and then on to Germany for the operation. As he rides in the Humvee, it dawns on the soldier that he is leaving the arena.

Sean will miss his buddies, but he also realizes that he will now have some decent food, the company of friendly and helpful U.S. Army Nurses and a return to the States to recover. He is relieved. Sean feels nearly no pain despite the fact that he has just been shot in the foot. He may require surgery and he was given only minimal pain medication.

Story Two: The Same Traumatic Injury with Considerable Pain

A 19-year-old young man, Mike, has spent three months in community college. He decides to go out with some friends for a burger and they end up in a fairly rough part of town. Mike notices that one of his friends is wearing a red baseball hat. Just as Mike starts to tell his friend to take off his hat, a shot is heard.

This neighborhood is rough territory and red represents membership to a particular gang. The shot pierces Mike's shoe and breaks his toe or metatarsal bone. He and his friends panic; they are fearful the shooter will return. Everyone scrambles to call for help. Mike is scared for his life. His pain is intense. All he wanted was a burger with his friends and now he has been randomly shot by someone who thought he was part of an opposing gang. Mike worries that he will have to miss his community school classes and that he does not have health insurance. He will probably have to have surgery at a county hospital, which is notorious for sub-par medical care.

When the paramedics arrive and bandage his wound, Mike is in a lot of pain. They give him a shot of morphine and he is off by ambulance to the local county hospital. In the emergency room, Mike has to wait for two hours to see a doctor while experiencing excruciating pain. He needs a lot more pain medication before the doctor will finally see him, review the x-rays and call to admit him for orthopedic surgery.

Looking at These Stories Side by Side

In both stories, the men suffer traumatic injuries. Yet one suffers little and the other experiences great pain. What is the key difference in their stories, which explains their different experiences?

In one scenario, the soldier needs no pain medicine and is excited and elated to be getting a "go home in one piece" ticket. On the other, the student's life is turned upside down, from health to injury, from school to disability, from solvency to medical bills.

The student Mike, with the same physical injury as the first, suffers far more pain. This phenomenon was first reported by Dr. Henry K. Beecher, an anesthetist in the Second World War. (10)

Why did they have such different experiences with pain even though the injury was the same? The context was very different in each case. We now understand that the natural pain killing systems of the body, *endorphins, enkephalins* and others, help the injured soldier to tolerate the physical trauma.

In the second case, fear, worry and anxiety in this unanticipated situation led to an exaggeration of the pain, not a reduction of it.

These stories illustrate this lesson:

Lesson Two: The context and the interpretation of the pain by the patient and its perceived significance are crucial.

How does the brain interpret the body's signals and how is it influenced by the context? The brain is not just passively accepting all the sensory information feeding to it like a computer's central processing unit (CPU).

What actually happens is that the brain is interpreting the meaning of these signals and reacting to them. Part of this reaction is emotional. The other part is nerve signals, which are sent from the brain down to the body that amplify or reduce the sensations.

If you believe your pain will never go away, or if you believe your pain is degenerative and no one can fix your pain, then that belief actually will affect your pain. Studies have shown that a patient's belief as to whether an antidepressant will or will not work is a key factor in the success of that medication. (11) Functional MRI studies and Q-EEG analyses of these depressed patients show that researchers can predict who will get better based on the blood flow to the frontal cortex of the brain.

Therefore, it appears that your belief causes changes in the *pre-frontal cortex* and *anterior cingulate gyrus* of the brain, which focuses attention on the pain or reduces that focus. I believe that this attention is part of a process of amplification that Dr. Sarno has previously described as "ischemia" or lack of oxygen flow to the tissues. This makes the pain persist and even intensify. (See Chapter V.)

On the other hand, if your pain is ultimately benign as it is in the case of TMS pain, then a belief that the pain **will** go away and that the pain is **not** due to structural damage will activate the appropriate pathways to make the pain go away.

Again, your recovery from pain depends upon on your understanding of the meaning, the context **and** the true diagnosis for the pain.

NERVE SIGNALS ARE A TWO-WAY STREET

Howard Fields, M.D., Ph.D., Neurologist and Researcher from UCSF, has elegantly demonstrated and described the nerve signals that leave the brain and go to the spinal cord and body. (12) Other researchers had always focused on the more well-known signals or sensations that come up from the body to the brain.

The mind/brain responds to the "mindless" sensory input from the nerves and uses the interpretation from the higher brain functions. This means that the context in which the pain occurred and the understanding of why it is there modifies the response to the pain, the perception of the pain and the physiology of the affected organ by *efferent* signals, which are signals from the brain sent down to the body.

This process is not widely discussed in the medical literature, as its significance is clearly understood. But it is one of the key phenomena in explaining chronic pain. Understanding this process can help us to eliminate chronic pain.

Without the interpretation of the brain, a human is like a robot or a machine that cannot respond to signals from the body. But with this deepened understanding of how pain is perceived, one becomes a complex nervous system, a whole person.

The person inside us has the life experiences, the emotional reactions, the memories and the values that determine how the pain will be interpreted and whether the pain will be amplified, suppressed or disappear completely.

This deeper understanding of how chronic pain works is a critical piece of information that is often missed by much of the medical profession, as well as the alternative community. I educate a person to pay attention to the emotions, context, and meaning of the injury which helps them to ease their pain on their own. This is a highly effective tool that I teach.

The lesson is here. You are not a passive player in your pain experience. What you believe, what you know, what you feel and what you do are crucial to changing and often eliminating, your persistent pain pattern. Hence another Lesson:

Lesson Six: Pain (sensory) signals are a two-way street. The mind/brain plays a crucial role in what you feel.

The signals are going "north" to the brain and "south" to the body. The body hurts less, if at all, once the patient assumes some control over the process. The control may mean self-talk, journaling, psychotherapy, exercise and release of fear and grief. It is the doing, rather than being passive, that is crucial to eliminating the pain.

Try this. Start telling yourself that you are in control of the pain and that the pain is not going to rule your life anymore. This may seem silly at first, but self-talk is the mechanism by which we change the chatter in our brain into a re-programming message for our "software" up there. Come up with a phrase like, "This pain is in my control. Go away!" to affirmatively indicate your belief in control over the pain. Repeat the phrase to yourself many times a day. This begins the re-programming of the central nervous system.

PREOCCUPATION WITH PAIN

Some people with neck and low back pain or tension headaches are unintentionally preoccupied with the signals or sensations emanating from their neck, back or head. Other people might easily ignore these nerve signals or naturally minimize them. However, the mind/brain of a person experiencing the pain may amplify these nerve signals by consciously focusing on them.

I see this all the time in my office. Some people, especially perfectionists and worriers, are extremely focused on their bodies. They need a lot of reassurance about their health. One young man, in his late 20s, comes to mind. He came to see me with a folder that was unusually thick for a basically healthy man of his age. It was stuffed full of his prior lab tests, x-ray reports, nerve testing and many assessments from other doctors. He had concerns about his pain and, despite a totally normal examination and benign diagnoses from a variety of specialists, it took a lot of work, including counseling, to help him resolve his problem.

In this case, the counseling started with my usual office consultation and follow-up visits. It continued with psychotherapy with one of the mental health practitioners to whom I refer patients. He did well with treatment, but continues to have low-level symptoms due to an underlying personality makeup that drives him to worry and, one might say, obsess about his condition(s).

There are different reasons why some people tend to focus on their pain and thereby amplify it. One is genetic susceptibility. Some pain conditions, including a tendency for chronic pain, do run in families. However, I still find this type of pain can be successfully treated, whether its origins are biological or cultural.

WHY WHAT YOU THINK YOU KNOW
ABOUT PAIN IS WRONG

Unfortunately, during an acute attack, some people allow their minds to run wild on hunches, fears and bad information. Sometimes patients assume the worst and, in the process of worrying about pain, they actually make it worse. Many health professionals make the problem more severe when they tell their patients, who are suffering a routine acute attack, of all the things that *could* be wrong. This only intensifies fear and causes patients to seek all sorts of "solutions" that literally run from A to Z, such as: *acupuncture, Botox injections, chiropractic, deep tissue massage, electrical stimulation, facet blocks, growth hormone, herbs and hypnosis, injections, joint mobilization, k-laser, ligament injections, magnets, medications and meditation, narcotics, osteopathy, physical therapy, qi-gong, reiki healing or Rolfing, surgery, TENS units (and other electrical nerve stimulation), ultrasound treatments, Vax-D (a form of traction), water therapy, and yoga.* (I am still trying to find the back pain solution that starts with a Z. I'm sure someone, somewhere, is working on it.)

New solutions seem to pop-up every year, with each methodology claiming to be the one that will finally solve the problem. Every time the pharmaceutical companies develop new pills and medications, it gives people great hope, hope that is usually short-lived, due to side effects, unfortunate drug interactions, high costs and ultimately the limited relief.

Even if a drug could be developed to undo chronic pain, would it not be better to first explore an approach that does not require taking a medication daily or perhaps forever — *first?* Should not doctors and patients work together to heal pain in a natural, holistic way, whenever possible? It is time to reconnect the mind and body, which have only recently, in an historical sense, been split apart in our Western conception of health and disease.

What is the answer? Who will solve this problem of unrelenting pain? Who will invent a new pill, shot or device to relieve it? You and millions of other patients with chronic pain are waiting for these answers. To date, no purely technological solution has ever appeared.

What if the solution is not a pill, shot or device at all? What if the explanation to your chronic pain is something that you can learn from the educational program that is described in this book? What if the answer ultimately lies in how *you* use your mind and brain to reevaluate and eradicate your pain with thought?

THINK AWAY YOUR PAIN

WHY WHAT YOUR DOCTOR TELLS YOU
ABOUT PAIN IS OFTEN WRONG

Here is an idea to ponder: Perhaps the reason your pain has not been resolved is that the approaches and models to which you have been exposed are inadequate or incorrect. Have any of them worked for you personally? Think about what you have tried so far.

Start by listing the treatments, the time involved, the practitioners you have seen and the money you have spent. If none of your treatments have worked more than temporarily, could it be because their treatment models are incorrect or incomplete? How much more time and more money will you spend before you begin to seek a different kind of understanding?

For many patients, I am the doctor of last resort. Patients come to see me nearly every week and describe how they have spent thousands of dollars, out of pocket, on a variety of medical and alternative treatments, all without any real pain relief. Some treatments help for a while, others do nothing at all and still others make the problem worse, but still cost a lot!

Remarkably, for almost all of these pain sufferers, no doctor has ever asked them about their life, their feelings, their worries and their fears. Patients are asked about injuries, pain history, medications and previous treatments. Many tests are typically ordered. But the diagnoses are all too often based solely on these test results.

SEEING THE PERSON WITH PAIN

Unfortunately, what these doctors never seem to notice is the *person* suffering from the pain. Each person has a unique narrative, an individual story that is often the key to understanding why the pain began. This narrative will help them to find relief. The current healthcare system provides incentives for every kind of treatment, except the concept of simply sitting, talking to patients and getting to know them as unique persons in pain.

Interestingly, the ancients understood the mind's influence on pain long ago. We are just now rediscovering what they learned. Consider the history of the term psychosomatic. Early physicians could trace a connection between people who had healthy thoughts who felt better than those people with dark thoughts and worries. Today, we call this mind-body medicine. It is the same basic idea that a health problem, such as pain, can be created by the mind.

The words psychosomatic or psycho-physiological are highly misunderstood, both by doctors and by patients. Patients often assume that their condition is being described as fake or phony. They feel that they are being accused of crazy behavior or exaggerating their pain. Too often, doctors use the diagnosis as a label to categorize patients that they do not like. Doctors do not take the time to understand the patient, especially when they cannot treat them with their usual set of tools: the prescription pad and the scalpel.

To me, the term psychosomatic is **basic science** and a crystal clear philosophy, as well. Psyche and soma, mind and body, are the integrated parts of a human being. You cannot have one without the other in a healthy, functioning person.

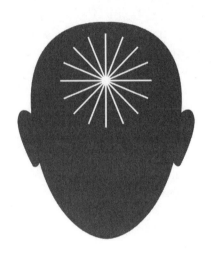

CHAPTER III

Why Do You Have Pain?

All of us have experienced pain in different degrees through-out our lives. For most of us, pain is a natural and healthy way that our bodies warn us we are doing something that is hurting us. In most cases pain serves its purpose well.

Understanding why we experience pain is part of learning to cope with it. Studies have shown that when we think about our pain negatively, we actually hurt more. (1) It is our nature as human be-ings to assume the worst and believe the pain that we are suffering indicates something is seriously wrong. Fortunately, that is usually not the case. By the time you finish reading this chapter you will see that:

• Pain is signaling a temporary issue with our bodies. Pain is not the warning sign of a major problem.

• Pain is frustrating to people because it can be difficult to get over, even after the body has largely healed itself.

• Pain is a challenge to cope with as an adult, in part due to the way we learned how to handle pain when we were younger.

• Pain is striking people who are living a modern lifestyle of hectic work schedules and difficult professional demands.

• Pain is becoming worse due to quirks or unique aspects of our personalities that serve to intensify pain by channeling our stress into the body.

THE REAL CAUSES OF PAIN

What is the experience of pain? A simple answer is that you feel pain because your brain receives distress signals from the nerves in a particular part of your body. A more sophisticated answer might include the process, in the mind/brain, under some circumstances, of amplifing, rather than ignoring, minor sensory signals from the body. Furthermore, the brain is able to send signals back to the body that can relieve or cause pain. (2) Your brain is the captain of your nervous system, the central processor of the bodily computer and the controller of your movements, sensations and mood. In Chapter VI, you will learn the research data that document how the brain can generate pain, seemingly out of nowhere.

Why would your brain want *you* to feel pain? The "you" here is your mind or the thinking conscious part of the nervous system. Let us look at two theories.

• Pain as a Structural Problem. The brain is trying to warn you of ongoing damage to the body, as is the case of a wound, burn or fracture. It could also be a growing tumor, a compressed or inflamed nerve, a swollen bursa, or a torn tendon or ligament. These are the things that can be spotted by a trained physician on an examination x-ray, ultrasound or MRI. These are the instances where the brain knows that action needs to be taken and therefore the alert, pain, is turned on.

• Pain as a Mind/Brain Problem. When the brain amplifies or creates sensations that do not represent bodily damage but are experienced as bodily sensations, pain is a mind-body problem. In terms of its cause, this pain, while subjectively indistinguishable from the first type, is more of a brain phenomenon than a bodily problem. To look at this further is one of the keys to understanding your chronic pain and to innovative successful ways of treating it.

Lesson One: The source of chronic pain is often the nervous system and brain, not structural injury.

MIND/BRAIN AND MIND-BODY

The mind/brain is a concept that I will refer to often in this book, especially in this chapter. That is why it is important to have a deeper understanding of what I mean.

When I refer to the mind/brain, I am describing how both thinking and feeling occur as brain functions, which, as a concept, we describe as our "mind." One definition of the mind is the element that enables a person to be aware of the world and their experiences and to think and to feel. The mind is the faculty of consciousness and thought. (3) I use the term mind/brain to demonstrate the physical reality of mind as embodied in the brain.

I do not intend a philosophical discussion on the definition of the mind. What I do want to convey is that cognition and emotions can be thought of as originating in the brain. The brain is part of the body and it is the nerve center of the body. I use the term mind/brain to emphasize and clarify the direct connection of the actual neural pathways, along with brain and nervous system signaling, that account for chronic pain and our innate ability to control or eliminate it. The reality of this linkage, or unity, allows the otherwise abstract concepts of thought, feelings and even psychology, to be understood more concretely. The mind and emotions are as real as your arm and they are embodied in the brain. This is the mind/brain.

By moving away from the conceptual split between mind and brain, we can grasp the concreteness of how our brain works and how our mind/brain can control the body. I also want you to see the whole of your "expanded"' body as one. Therefore, even the title

45

of this book begins to carry deeper meaning. *Think Away Your Pain.* Understand that thinking is part of the brain, as well as affecting the brain. The brain is part of the body and it affects the body!

The concept of a split between the body and the mind is historically and culturally based. "Cartesian Duality," the term from the French philosopher Rene Descartes, refers to the split between mind and body. The reason for this splitting of the two is complex and has historical and religious components.

Here is where I feel Dr. John Sarno's contribution to our understanding of the mind-body link is so important. One cannot understand pain without reconnecting these splits. Dr. Sarno began this process, in a powerful way, with the writing that he began in the late 1970's on this subject. He produced four books. His clinical work cared for and cured tens of thousands of patients. (4-7)

I have long used the term mind-body or MindBody in some of my prior writing to designate the linkage between the mind and what is happening in the rest of our body. The hyphen represents that linkage or connection. Using the two capitalized words together, without a space or hyphen, emphasizes the tightness of this linkage and graphically highlights the vital importance of **both** parts of the linkage. Other authors have continued this same format since I first started using it.

FREUDIAN PSYCHOLOGY

Concepts in our treatment of chronic pain, which have led to current TMS treatments, are derived in part from some of the older Freudian-derived theories of the mind and psychology. Freudian psychology first made us aware of the unconscious mind and the depth of our internal emotional lives. Brain research has taken this theory further to show us how different parts of the brain may function in ways akin to Freudian theories. (8) (9)

Followers of Freud's thinking have much in common with

the modern researchers who utilize high-powered tools to peer into our skulls to examine the brain. My focus is on integrating these traditional perspectives with up-to-date research on the brain. In some ways, at first glance, the older models are better descriptive models for patients and therapists. The newest research illustrates how laboratory science is beginning to unlock the mysteries of the brain that coincide with many, but not all, of the prior conclusions.

WHEN THERE IS AN ISSUE WITH THE BODY

There is no question in my mind that various structural conditions can cause pain. Two examples follow, one an injury and the other a rare spinal cord tumor. These examples will illustrate how to differentiate injury, or structural disease from the mind/brain generated chronic pain whose treatment is the subject of this book.

With structural injury or damage, the pain may be present constantly or most of the time. The pain you experience typically varies depending upon how the painful area is being moved or stretched. For example, with a torn knee ligament, the knee may not hurt when immobilized. With bursitis of the hip, pain often fades when the hip joint is not being used. Therefore, pain associated with a structural injury serves as a useful and important signal that you should not ignore.

STRUCTURAL PROBLEMS: AN EXAMPLE

The following is a rare case, but it illustrates some important points about pain that is caused by structural issues. Some fifteen years ago, a young man came to me complaining of unrelenting pain in his back and groin. Since he already had a reportedly normal MRI reviewed by a well-known surgeon, I found no reason not to try a mind-body approach when he came to me for relief. The patient did not improve with my treatment. The excruciating pain that kept him up at night did not abate. It was clear something was wrong.

Another MRI, this time performed with a slightly wider view of the spine, showed a spinal cord tumor. He was immediately hospitalized for neurosurgical removal of this mass and did well after that procedure.

My point in mentioning this rare cause for pain in this young man is that when there is a true structural condition, it is extremely appropriate for your brain to alert you with continued pain as a warning signal something is wrong and needs your attention. These ongoing signals enabled doctors to make the diagnosis and direct the young man to treatment that prevented the tumor from growing. The pain the young man felt in his back and groin area, though ultimately **perceived** in his central nervous system, i.e. his mind/brain, **originated** with signals that were sent up to the brain from nerve endings near the tumor.

No amount of mind-body treatment would have eliminated this pain because it was truly a structural issue. The remainder of this book will illustrate many different examples of pain that persists, despite being benign. This is pain that **both originates** and **is perceived** in the mind/brain and lacks a structural issue that requires surgical or even physical treatment.

TMS: A ROOT CAUSE OF PAIN

The nervous system is fallible and, in many chronic pain cases, it can be downright disingenuous. When working properly, the pain circuits in the nervous system serve to alert us that something is wrong and needs our attention, as was the case with the young man I just mentioned. With the kind of pain we are focusing upon in this book, the pain circuits are hijacked to serve a different and more mysterious purpose.

In these cases, the original threat is the emergence of a highly disturbing emotion, such as extreme rage, grief or shame, from the subconscious into consciousness. The emotional brain, whose structure we share with all other mammals, is relatively primitive and cannot distinguish the emergence of a threatening emotion from a real danger to our survival. All it can do is pass the warning, "There is a serious threat here," to the more sophisticated, higher-cognitive brain functions that decide what to do with it. Unfortunately, some of these higher-cognitive circuits are also subconscious and they can decide to take matters in their own hands without telling "the boss," the conscious higher-level cognitive circuits.

These circuits simply tell other brain functions, such as those that control muscle contraction and the dilation or constriction of blood vessels, to create a disturbance or distraction that will keep "the boss" too preoccupied to notice the "threat" of the emerging emotion. Hence the term I coined, "Distraction Pain Syndrome." (10)

Although the exact mechanisms may vary, some examples would be telling muscles to spasm persistently, causing a wicked attack of pain in the lower back, or telling blood vessels in the brain or its linings to constrict, as in a headache. In both examples the pain is very real and can be excruciating. The structures involved are not damaged; they are just functionally inappropriately, on a temporary basis. These sensations of pain are very real. The reason for the pain is not structural damage but the mind creating the pain. That is TMS. TMS can also be understood on the basis of brain mechanisms. (See Chapters VI and VIII.)

In most cases, the mind/brain somehow manages to deal with the problem, possibly consciously or more often, subconsciously. Typically the pain resolves within a few days or weeks. However, the pain can theoretically continue indefinitely, as long as it needs to keep the disturbing emotions under wraps. The longer it persists, the stronger the associated neural pathways become, leading to pain that can last for years or even decades in some extreme cases.

For example, a young father has lifted his three-year-old son countless times. One day, he lifts his son exactly the same way he always does, but does so during a period of his life when he has been fretting about losing a job promotion. This time, his back muscles, primed by the stress of his work situation, go into a painful spasm.

Because of his personality and his current work pressures, he might worry much more than a person who tends to be less hard on himself. He quite naturally begins to worry that something is wrong with his back. If the young father responds to this painful back attack with a lot of worry, fear and emotional *amplification*, the problem may persist for a week or even longer.

PAIN IS NO LONGER A WARNING, BUT THE PROBLEM ITSELF

It stands to reason that treatments based upon inaccurate or incomplete understanding of the condition will probably not be successful. The key issue here is to determine whether the pain is due to a structural issue or a mind/brain phenomenon. This decision will determine the appropriate treatment for the pain.

Deeper within the mind/brain of the young father, processes could occur that might favor the pain to continue, as the mind/brain may take advantage of this usually brief pain attack. While the initial pain signals are useful in telling his brain that he must rest briefly to relax his back, the mind/brain might also desire a few sick days that will allow him to avoid the stressful work environment. Or, if the emotions stirred up by the work situation are really threatening, he may come to feel safer to go on disability, the loss of income notwithstanding. These subconscious processes of mind/brain trickery can lead to chronic pain. They also explain why pain can still persist in the absence of a clear, structural cause.

Another explanation for why pain persists is that the brain may receive continuous, low-level signals from some part of the body, possibly a mildly arthritic joint or a tight neck muscle. But, instead of noting the nerve messages and suppressing or ignoring them, the mind/brain **amplifies** them.

An example of suppressing or reducing a sensation is our diminishing awareness of our buttocks when we sit on a chair. Initially, we note the firmness of the chair and assess it for comfort. Soon thereafter, our brain completely ignores those same sensations and we move on with reading, speaking or computing while sitting in that same chair. We may notice our bottom again, later, when we feel an urge to squirm, adjust, move or get up. This can happen in minutes or much longer, depending upon our interest in the activity. The design of our chair, the temperature and the comfort of our buttocks are sensations that we ignore.

We are not constantly aware of all sensory signals. Turning our awareness on and off is something our brain generally does well. But what happens when it fails, as it sometimes does?

If you are like most people who first learn how the brain can cause pain, you might be a bit skeptical. You assume you are the expert in what is going on, not some unconscious state of mind. But if you think about it, your body is constantly monitoring and conducting vital functions all day long while you are blissfully unaware. Consider our digestion. We are generally not thinking about the digestion processes going on in our thirty feet of small and large intestine unless something is wrong. And by something wrong I mean that we are hungry, something is not digesting well or we are feeling stressed.

While the brain gets plenty of sensory input, it knows what to ignore and what to focus upon. Sometimes, however, in relation to worry or excitement, our emotions get the best of us and we experience a nervous stomach, butterflies or diarrhea.

I find that an integrated mind/brain perspective brings us closer to the truth about chronic pain. The mind/brain approach is a way of keeping the pain sufferer focused on this broader perspective that is more scientifically accurate and practical in relieving chronic pain. Finally, this integrated mind/brain perspective leads us to a solution for the problem of chronic pain that both patients and health care professionals will find more useful and scientifically accurate.

CHANGING THE WAY YOU THINK
ABOUT YOUR PAIN

When something feels wrong in our bodies but there is no dis-ease or structural damage, the condition is properly called a *functional syndrome*. This means the conditions are real, painful or otherwise discomforting but are not problematic in terms of our health. These functional syndromes show no irreversible changes like a pathological disease might show.

Functional syndromes might sound like pretty obscure things, but they show up in rather common, and at times, unpleasant ways. Functional syndromes include tension headaches, jaw pain, irritable bowel syndrome, fibromyalgia, and yes, *myofascial* pain, all of which can be TMS.

In a functional syndrome, the symptoms are real, of course, but the change in the area of the body that is affected is not due to a localized, irreversible, permanent, structural pathology (the disease process) but rather to an ultimately benign, reversible, brain-triggered problem.

This way of understanding pain is hopeful and even exciting because the pain is fixable, not by surgery on the body, medication or even local treatment, but rather by changing how the brain responds so that it stops sending, amplifying or responding to pain signals in an exaggerated way. How this is accomplished will be discussed in detail later in this book.

TRAINING YOUR BRAIN TO STOP HURTING YOU

Your understanding of why you hurt may have been wrong all along and this may be limiting your ability to improve. This is such an important point that I am going to repeat it: **Your basic understanding of why you hurt may be wrong. This may be limiting your ability to improve.** The techniques and treatment approaches that follow require you to play an active role and to think differently.

Lesson Three: Psychology and education can change the mind/brain and cure pain, not just manage it.

Improvement requires a **change of mind**. This book will help you to understand the intricacies of pain. Then you can learn how to change your thinking. By altering how you deal with stress and tension and by changing the fear response to an "I understand and I am in control" response, the pain will improve.

The brain is very complex and incompletely understood. Pain that persists is more of a "brain pain" than a body pain in many cases. If you have "brain pain" (TMS), then your mind can affect the pain, change it and make it go away. There are well-defined mechanisms to explain why chronic pain is more complex but more treatable than one might expect. The source of the chronic pain is often the nervous system/brain not the area of your body in which you feel the pain nor where you suspect structural damage.

Lesson 1: The source of the chronic pain is often the nervous system and brain, not a structural injury.

YOUR CHILDHOOD MAY BE HURTING YOU NOW

The way you were brought up can have a huge effect on how you experience pain as an adult. (1) Understanding your past might be a key part of understanding why you are feeling pain now. When I ask patients about their childhood, their answers usually fall into one of a few categories, including:

• Pressure Cooker. One category involves people who describe a happy, loving childhood, but with tremendous pressure from parents who expected high-achievement from them. Lest we think it is always the parent's fault, I sometimes get the distinct impression that the patient who felt pressured while still a child is an innately driven person. Genetics, or "nature over nurture," may explain these differences in people.

• Dysfunctional Situations. Another category of answers includes individuals with more challenging childhoods, often involving families that were divorced and where drug issues, alcoholism and other addictions were part of the family situation. Patients with an alcoholic parent are affected for the rest of their life by the inconsistencies of that parent. These patients, whether afflicted with addiction themselves or not, need special nurturance and often good therapy to stay on track emotionally.

• Round Pegs in Square Holes. Still another category of childhood experience includes people who just did not quite fit in with their siblings and parents. They were different, perhaps do not have close relationships now and may have moved far away from their families of origin. It was nothing terrible, just a mismatch that led to a feeling of not belonging. This may lead to a desire to belong elsewhere or to a loneliness where that lack of a childhood connection makes future adult relationships more challenging. I am thinking now of a woman who grew up in a traditional Mennonite family. Her interests in art and photography were very different from those of her family and the culture of her upbringing. She found these differences hard to reconcile and that led to loneliness and eventual estrangement from her family.

54

• Cruel Upbringing. The most challenging group to treat are the individuals who experienced a cruel childhood with emotional or physical abuse, sexual molestation or abandonment. People whose experiences fit into this category can be successfully treated, but treatment is usually longer. Good psychotherapy is usually required to help advance the healing. Even if they have been in therapy before, I usually incorporate a specialized TMS therapist in their treatment process.

Understanding my patient's childhood is the first step toward helping them to understand the connection between their life story and their pain. As they tell me the history of their pain, I listen to the life that weaves its way in and around the story of symptoms, treatments and procedures. This narrative is a key to understanding the pain, diagnosing TMS and unraveling its web of confusion.

HOW CHILDREN LEARN TO AMPLIFY PAIN

Another reason for a brain's particular reaction to sensation might be how the patient was raised as a child to react to and deal with pain. Parents respond differently to a child in pain. In some families, a hug and a pat, along with a "go out and play now, dear" may work wonders to minimize a child's concern over pain.

However, some parents, even with the best of intentions, may excessively focus on the child's complaints of pain, be it a headache, tummy pain or a skinned knee. Whether conscious or not, this can lead the child to getting what he wants, such as parental attention, time off school, missing soccer practice or avoiding a dreaded party. The fulfillment of this desire then reinforces the mind/brain pain connection to a detrimental effect.

I recall a patient of mine who as a teenager was very shy about attending parties and social gatherings. Just before he was supposed to be ready to go, he often got a stomach ache. His family became used to these pains and allowed him to stay home to recover from his "virus" or "food poisoning." Eventually he outgrew the anxiety, but it would have been better to deal with the underlying stress and tension by helping him understand, express and address his fears.

In general, a better way to deal with children having medically benign pain is to sit down and explore the child's feelings about school, friends, bullies and other pressures. By bridging the mind/brain gap that often underlies these complaints, we can help our children better understand their stress. I am convinced that teaching kids from an early age to see pain as a warning, that something else is bothering them, would prevent a lot of future health conditions and chronic pain. The younger the better, I believe, when it comes to exposing people to these concepts in an age appropriate way.

The Children's Hospital of Pennsylvania (CHOP) calls this issue "Amplified Musculoskeletal Pain Syndrome" (AMPS). Their recommendations are similar to ours, although perhaps a little more behaviorally focused. (11)

HOW WORK CAUSES PAIN

Over and over I hear from people that their pain started just after an emotional crisis or during a period of prolonged grief. More commonly, pain begins in relation to their work. When the pain is due to a job, it is often related to an uncomfortable situation with a supervisor or co-worker.

People also get stuck in jobs that are not right for them. Some people must contend with a boss who is overly controlling or abusive. There is a natural desire for stability and people often resist the only ultimate solution, which is finding a new job, launching a new career or at least seeking a transfer. Sometimes there are family or financial pressures that make a job change nearly impossible.

There is a lot of research about back pain in industry and much of it leads to the same conclusions. Job dissatisfaction is a significant contributor to pain. (12) In fact, negative feelings toward work are a bigger risk factor for an unresolved back injury than abnormal x-rays or weak abdominal muscles. So if you have a job you hate, getting a new one will likely help ease your pain much more than just about anything else.

Patients who are ambivalent about the kind of work they do are faced with a different type of emotional stress. I see musicians who are stuck making mortgage loans and social reformers unhappy in clerical positions. These conflicts create internal tensions that can manifest in pain. The pain often begins just after a severe emotional crisis such as a death or breakup of a relationship. But pain also flares up at the point in a job or relationship where a person feels stuck with nowhere to go.

Lesson Two: The context and the interpretation of the pain by the patient and its perceived significance are crucial.

It is the interaction between the external stress and the internal personality makeup that creates the pain. Of the two, sometimes it is easier to change the external, such as changing jobs, ending a relationship and rethinking a career.

Often, however, the clearest and most important change we can make is within ourselves. We do not attempt to change our personality, which is probably impossible and certainly extremely difficult as well as time consuming. Instead, we attempt to modify how we react to the stressor and understand more clearly our motivations, fears and anger. This is usually enough to help break the cycle of pain.

YOUR PERSONALITY AND YOUR PAIN

Probing deeper into a particular patient's chronic pain condition requires following a two-track approach:

1) Seek out pertinent medical information.

2) Seek out pertinent psychological information.

This is the key to making the correct diagnosis and therefore being able to successfully treat the otherwise confusing chronic pain conditions.

Assessing Personality: In terms of finding out about a patient's personality, I will ask:

Are you a perfectionist?

Are you a people pleaser?

Are you hard on yourself?

Are you highly responsible for others?

Are you sensitive to criticism?

By asking these questions and observing the response, I determine whether a person with pain is a "Type T" personality.

TYPE T PERSONALITY

Many years ago, I began to refer to the constellation of personality traits often found in mind-body sufferers as the "Type T" personality. This was an opportunity to expand upon on the nomenclature first described by Drs. Meyer and Friedman for people with heart disease as the "Type A" personality. (13) (14) Type T gave a name to some of what Dr. Sarno had first described. (4) (5)

In the Type T personality, "T" is for "tension." A Type T personality refers to someone who is tension prone and therefore more

58

susceptible to mind-body disorders. Patients, and sometimes their accompanying spouses, can tell the physician whether they have these qualities or tendencies. They usually share with me that doctors do not tend to ask about these highly relevant aspects of their psycho-social history.

When I talk to patients about their personality characteristics, I want to understand their risk factors for mind-body conditions. I am also looking to understand the patient at a deeper level than usual. A superficial understanding of a patient leads to a generic or "one size fits all" diagnosis. A deeper understanding of the patient as a person leads to a customized, personalized diagnosis and treatment approach. It takes a little more time and attention on the doctor's part, but it is worth it in the end.

By gaining a deeper understanding of the patient's personality, I will explain later in the visit how personality is relevant to their pain and how an awareness of these traits and tendencies can lead us to a therapeutic program that involves moderating some of these extremes.

THE ALPHABET SOUP FOR TYPE T WOULD BE:

M motivated, achiever

N nice, a goodist is someone who is driven to perform good acts

O prefers order, not necessarily orderly

P perfectionist, a people pleaser

Q quick to judge

R responsible

S self-critical, one who is hard on oneself

T Type T

In order to be a Type T, you need one or two characteristics in force, not all five or seven. Many of my patients exhibit or admit to characteristics such as these:

- Hard on Oneself

- People Pleaser

- Responsible. Goodist. Perfectionist, or 'closet' perfectionist

Very few have all of the characteristics in the list. That is not a requirement for diagnosis, nor is it common.

MANAGING YOUR TYPE T PERSONALITY

Do you have to change your personality to succeed in my treatment approach? Can you even do this?

The answers I give patients are NO and NOT THAT MUCH. As one looks deeper to understand the roots of these traits, I do discuss learning how **to tune down** some of the overly powerful aspects of one's personality.

Type T people are hard on themselves, highly responsible and concerned about the perceptions of others. In the office, I discuss with these patients how to turn down the dial on their perfectionism from 9.5 to an 8, on a scale of 1 to 10. I describe lowering the volume of responsibility from 9 to perhaps 7.5. By these adjustments, I mean to illustrate to patients that relatively small changes, that we can control, can go a long way toward reducing the pressure and consequently the pain.

They do not have to go from Type T to Type B. At its extreme, Type B's are ultra-mellow, insensitive, irresponsible individuals. The proverbial beach bum? Instead, Type T's just need to be more aware of the way they respond, so that they can learn to gear it down a notch or two.

When these individuals work with one of the psychotherapists to whom I refer for mind-body therapy, they learn to understand how these Type T personality traits form. They learn to address some of the self-esteem issues and unmet emotional needs that often underlie them.

Personality matters. The "illness" we have is shaped and in some cases created, by the person that we are. The one size fits all model of healthcare may be efficient, like fast food that is not very nutritious and is clearly not specific to an individual's particular dietary needs.

Taking the additional time to know the patient and using that information to understand their pain condition is vitally important in the successful treatment of these disorders.

TAKE HOME POINTS:

Think about your own personality and list the Type T personality characteristics that you notice in yourself. Are you a perfectionist, a people pleaser, highly responsible and hard on yourself? How does this affect you in dealing with people, stress and tension?

Do you feel that doctors have looked at your pain in a highly individualized way or have you been treated more generically as a disease entity? Think about how that approach in your case fails to provide a clear path for healing.

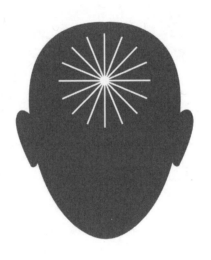

CHAPTER IV

Types of Pain

Structural Causes and Mind-Body Causes

Most of the causes of pain are not nearly as irreversible as you might believe or fear. Even persistent pain you have been dealing with for years can often go away once you figure out what has been bothering you.

With that said, there are some situations when your pain is not caused by your mind, but a structural issue with your body. In my experience many of these cases are fairly easy to diagnose in this day and age. With modern medical techniques, including magnetic resonance imaging (MRI), it is actually the mind-body disorders that are missed, not the rare structural malformation that you might hear about on TV shows.

This book is all about helping you understand that it is often not your body, but your mind/brain, that is causing or perpetuating your pain. A big part of making that connection is finally accepting that there is nothing structurally wrong with your body. Even if your mind is causing your problems, it is important to rule out the structural conditions that can exist.

This chapter is not here to scare you. In fact, I am loath to even include it, because it might make some people, who do not have any structural problems, start to diagnose and convince themselves that they do. It is prudent and necessary to go see a doctor, making sure he or she examines you for these unusual conditions.

Before you can accept the solutions to pain in this book, you need to completely sign on to the concept that your body is sound. The best way to accomplish this is through a thorough evaluation by a trained medical professional who is experienced with spotting physical problems, but ideally one who does not over-emphasize minor physical issues. If nothing is found, then through the process of elimination, you can start to understand that if your body is not hurting you, it must be your mind/brain.

WHY CHECKING WITH YOUR DOCTOR IS IMPORTANT

If you just got hurt, maybe you are the optimistic type who thinks it will go away in a relatively short period of time. In the vast majority of cases, that is true. The human body is remarkably good at repairing itself. But when pain starts lasting a little too long, that is when the danger of chronic pain sets in.

Your first stop in seeing what is causing your pain should be a doctor that can find structural sources of pain. Examples include a broken arm, a spinal cord tumor, severe nerve impingement, cancer or gout. A physical examination and appropriate testing, usually including a simple x-ray, ultrasound or advanced CT or MRI scan, can accomplish this as long as it is appropriately determined by a physician who is skilled in interpretation and who is sensitive to your overall pain syndrome.

The way doctors deal with early chronic pain follows from its cause. Here are some causes that a doctor considers:

• **Structural.** There can be structural issues with the body that result in pain. A mass, growth, tumor, severe infection or nerve pressing against a bone are all examples of structural problems. These conditions are pretty rare. For some conditions, structural treatment means that surgery, antibiotics or other procedures are required to solve the problem. Other structural conditions, that involve inflammation or partial tears of a tendon or muscle, may require physical therapy or strengthening exercises. In some cases, injections may be appropriate. A hip *bursitis* or rotator cuff *tendonitis* can often respond very quickly to an injection of a cortico-steroid medication like Triamcinolone. These injections often address inflammation in the affected region.

• **Inflammatory/Chemical.** Rheumatoid arthritis, Polyarteritis and Lupus are all illnesses where pain results from inflammation. The treatment is typically chemical or pharmacological (medicine). Since inflammation is the problem, the treatment and goal is to reduce the inflammation and seek out its source. Emotional factors can certainly play a role, but a quick and often effective initial route to treating these conditions, before they damage the organ systems involved, is with powerful anti-inflammatory treatments. These might include Remicade, which is a potent medication that affects the immune response, for rheumatoid arthritis or inflammatory bowel disease.

• **Metabolic.** Your body is a remarkable cocktail of chemicals. The balance between sugars and acids must be in balance or problems can occur. When there is a problem with your body's metabolic makeup, the treatment is to improve the metabolic pathways. For gout, the cause is uric acid deposition (deposits in joints) and the treatment is often to reduce the uric acid in the blood and increase excretion (removal) by the kidneys.

But chronic pain **often** does not fall into one of these neat checkboxes. Many cases exist where the sources of pain are not structural, chemical or metabolic. The lack of these clear diagnostic categories often cause many doctors to throw up their hands and chalk up your pain to the inexplicable. Others may think that remedies for structural problems, while not appropriate, may work because they have worked on other patients that did have structural issues. Or they may focus on very minor structural changes, such as a bulging disc, that are actually equally prevalent in those with no symptoms at all! (1)

Unfortunately, while this gives the doctor a diagnosis to tell you and write on his billing slip, it often gives your unconscious a year's worth of worry to undo. Sometimes longer.

After ruling out structural problems, the next step **should** be the exploration of emotional factors and issues. A focus is needed on the huge power of emotional, psychological and mental solutions to affect health and initiate healing. Unfortunately, the vast majority of physicians, chiropractors and other medical professionals will never get to this step. They do not feel comfortable with this process or do not have the training or insight to help in this arena. (See Chapters XI and XII.)

CHANGING THE CONVERSATION
FROM THE BODY TO THE MIND

When I first see patients, they are used to hearing the language of the body, for example, the spine and the back. Many have been to chiropractors, and some know the skeleton like the back of their own hand by staring at the skeletal models that are so commonly found in orthopedic and chiropractic offices.

After I have made a diagnosis of TMS and Mind-Body pain, then I start talking to the patient in a new language.

The new language we begin to speak together is the language of the mind, the emotions and the brain. That transition occurs as I recap or rephrase the story they have told me of the chronology of their condition. I call this their narrative.

Understanding deepens during our conversation. As the patient questions me, they make additional connections to emotional issues and triggers that they now realize were tied to the onset or continuation of the pain. We also discuss their current relationships, or absence of same, and this often brings up other links.

Successful patients ultimately learn to change the narrative, to change the story of their pain and their life. The story becomes about how the pain started when I lost my job or when my boyfriend left me, rather than **just** about the softball game injury or the fall on the ice. This change is a crucial part of the healing process. (Chapter X)

PAIN CAUSED BY THE MUSCLES, SPINE AND MIXED CAUSES

Many of the discomforts that humans endure are easily explained. The common cold, while not curable, is at least understood by science as a virus. Influenza, which can be uncomfortable and even fatal in extremely rare cases, is brought to us by another type of virus.

Pain often lacks that simple cause. Many things can cause pain. Two people with similar pain in the exact same place might trace the cause to two completely different issues or triggers. It is this diversity in the locations, triggers and types of pain that makes diagnosis especially challenging for doctors.

Another way to categorize pain is to divide it among structural causes, mind/brain causes and mixed causes. Because most doctors are trained in structural diagnoses, they often throw their hands up at mind/brain causes, even if they have a clue that it is the underlying issue. As to mixed causes, forget about it!

The odds that your chronic pain is purely structural are low if you are reading this book. Why? Because for those with a simple structural explanation, patients have typically and appropriately received treatment before seeking out this kind of expanded, in-depth explanation of pain. These folks have improved on their own, with treatment or in spite of treatment, typically in four to six weeks or less.

So, what are some of the pain generators that could explain acute or chronic pain?

• **Issues with the Spine.** The spine is a stack of vertebrae carefully aligned in a column. These vertebrae are balanced on top of each other and need to be strong and rigid enough to support a standing human being. The spine remains flexible because of the ligaments that hold it together, the joints in the vertebrae and the discs that cushion between bones.

A culprit for pain in some cases is discs. Discs are flexible cushions between the vertebrae. In some cases, these discs can become weakened or injured and then bulge out severely to push on a nerve. It is important to note, though, that studies of people without back pain have shown many disc bulges, so use of this explanation requires a keen sensitivity to the extent of the structural issues seen on a MRI, compared to the patient's symptoms and physical exam findings, in the context of that patient's personality and emotional state. Recently, I had a patient with a small bulge to the right whose pain was in the left buttocks. The diagnosis was totally 100% TMS.

• **Spinal and Foraminal (Nerve Canal) Stenosis.** There are cases, usually in older individuals, where the spine goes through gradual changes over many years that results in the tunnels and canals, where the nerves enter and exit, becoming uncomfortably tight. Sometimes the vertebrae shift significantly causing this problem. Other times it is bone spurs. Rarely, small operations to widen these tunnels are helpful to give the nerves more room. Even more rare, larger operations that involve instrumentation and realignment of bones are required.

Stenosis of any kind, central or foraminal, must also be carefully evaluated because in early stages, it is an example of a change akin to gray hair that comes with aging, and therefore, of no significance. In advanced cases, however, it may be the cause of leg or arm pain, especially with exertion.

• **Muscles in the Back of the Body.** If you see a cross-section of a person's back, you may be surprised by the number and size of the muscles. Some people experience pulled muscles, sprains and spasms in the back or other parts of their body. These events can be painful and even result in bruising or lack of movement. There is also a belief that if muscles become strong or weak in an asymmetrical way, it can increase the odds of a muscle issue. Rather than a more severe or structural condition, muscle spasm and tightness are a common cause of acute back pain and is part of the chronic pain/ TMS syndrome.

The *piriformis* muscle can be especially tricky due to its position near the sciatic nerve. "Muscular sciatica" is caused by spasm of the piriformis muscle, often intermittently irritating the adjacent sciatic nerve. There are injection treatments for this; there are also stretching exercises that can loosen the muscle. If the problem persists, TMS is another cause of this spasm.

• **Joints.** Places where bones come together can be problematic in some cases. Joints in the hip are also to blame in some cases. Hip and knee joints can develop wear and tear. Sometimes they hurt. Occasionally the wear is more severe. The diagnosis of osteoarthritis and its treatment moves to the physical, by strengthening muscles and injecting various substances. In extreme cases, the bone and cartilage is replaced with an artificial joint.

• **Extremely Rare Situations.** Broken vertebrae, after an accident, can cause issues. Cancer in the back, again extremely rare, can be a legitimate reason why the doctor might diagnose something structural. The cancer can be primary or *metastatic* from its origins in the prostate or breast. MRI imaging will show this quite clearly.

INTERPRETING MRIS: WHAT TO LOOK FOR

Scared yet? If you read the section above you might already be diagnosing yourself with all sorts of horrible problems. Again, I can assure you, that if you are like a vast majority of the patients I see for chronic back pain, none of the factors above are present in your body. Even if they were, that does not mean any of these things are behind the pain that you are experiencing.

How can I be so sure about this? Modern imaging techniques. New ways to peer inside the human body were supposed to make it crystal clear, once and for all, what causes pain. MRIs and other scans were supposed to help doctors instantly pinpoint that gnarled spine or torn muscle so the repair could begin.

But you know what? Instead of helping doctors find what is wrong, it helped them to see what is not wrong. Rather than finding broken bodies and crooked vertebrae in back pain sufferers, MRIs for most people come back showing only normal variants. Again, it is akin to gray hair or the aging of the spine.

Rather than showing us what is wrong with the human body and clarifying the cause of pain, modern imaging helps us determine that the problem is not always with our bodies, but elsewhere. Knowing this totally changes the game when it comes to dealing with pain.

Do not take my word for it. According to a team of co-authors at the Clinical Efficacy Assessment Subcommittee of the American College of Physicians in 2007, 85% of the people that go to the doctor following an acute episode of back pain do not have any specific cause or disease. (2) Study after study has shown that there is rarely, if ever, an identifiable cause of the pain. The doctors found that actual structural problems are quite rare. Herniated discs were only present in fewer than 4% of the cases and spinal infection in only 0.01%.

The doctors pointed out the conditions that might warrant a closer look. Trouble with bowel or bladder function may be a sign of severe neurological issues. Sudden and extreme weight loss or back pain repeatedly waking a patient from sleep are signs. These are the **red flags** that doctors are trained to look for in relation to back pain. Fortunately, these flags are rarely flown.

So if it is not the body causing the pain for most of us, what is? The doctors found "Psychosocial factors and emotional distress should be assessed because they are stronger predictors of low back pain outcomes than either physical examination findings or severity and duration of pain." (2) Rather than telling physicians to examine MRIs, they are urging them to look into emotional factors as being the most likely source of pain, or at least, the reason the pain is not going away.

These doctor-researchers found that things like job dissatisfaction and depression can result in back pain. They wrote, "Evidence is currently insufficient to recommend optimal methods for assessing psychosocial factors and emotional distress." They found, too, that endless imaging and other tests of the body "usually cannot identify a precise cause, do not improve patient outcomes and incur additional expenses." (2)

WHY DOCTORS DO NOT KNOW ABOUT TMS

The medical profession is well-trained to detect and treat severe disease. Most doctors are good at what they do. They are technically skilled and know how to treat and what to prescribe once they diagnose. The problem is that the TMS diagnosis is not well known or well understood by the majority of medical doctors. Therefore, their list of diagnoses is lacking a very important one: mind/brain pain or TMS.

An anecdote that proves this point comes from an annual conference of the American College of Physicians that I attended in San Diego in 2007. I attended the conference as an exhibitor, along with my colleague Dr. Arthur P. Smith, Foundation Coordinator for the Seligman Medical Institute (SMI). SMI is a non-profit organization that provided funding for me to explore research into the mind-body approach. The institute provides support for the awareness and education of physicians in this diagnosis and method.

SMI decided to reserve a booth at this conference, which would be attended by thousands of internists. There were hundreds of booths. Drug companies sponsored most. The National Institutes of Health was represented. Other booths included military recruiters and various hospitals seeking doctors. Thousands of physicians were in attendance, and many stopped at our booth. They chatted with us and picked up a pen or a stress ball. (Get it?!) However, few, if any, were familiar with the groundbreaking work of Dr. John E. Sarno.

Clearly, the TMS diagnosis is not in the mainstream and many physicians have not even heard of it. While we talked to hundreds of doctors, mostly briefly, and handed out over a thousand flyers explaining our research and the diagnosis, we received only two phone or email responses, a terribly low ratio given the topic and conference.

Why are most doctors so reticent to learn about TMS? There are a number of reasons, including:

1) Lack of Support from Major Organizations. The diagnosis has not received the approval of any major specialty organization such as rheumatology, physical medicine, psychiatry or orthopedics. This creates a vicious circle of physician skepticism, lack of support and disinterest.

2) Limited Research Data. Most of the TMS success has been in real-life, not in clinical trials or lab data. Little research has been published to date and essentially none of that has been a randomized clinical trial (RCT), the so-called gold standard in research. (See Chapter XI.)

Why no research data? For one thing, research is expensive and drug companies are not interested in funding an approach that is non-pharmacological at its core and does not require medications. Research at a high level requires an infrastructure with a big operation of staff, computers, research assistants and testing equipment.

For another, funding from the National Institutes of Health (NIH) depends on connections, past history of publication, university affiliation and the support of fellow researchers. This tight club is difficult to break into and tends to study and reinforce what is already known and accepted, rather than approaching innovative new methodology and conceptualizations. (3) In comparison to academically based research, clinician researchers are also under-supported by funding at the NIH. (4)

Finally, I asked a research colleague if he had any idea why we had been turned down repeatedly at a prestigious university for a well-designed brain imaging study related to this treatment approach to pain. He answered, "I heard from the director that he was uncomfortable using **his** center for a study about an approach that wasn't widely accepted or mainstream." We wondered, "Isn't that how science progresses? Isn't testing non-mainstream methods the way to determine if they should become mainstream or fall by the way side?" Is Galileo rolling over in his grave as I write this?

SOLVING MIND-BODY PAIN IS NOT LUCRATIVE

3) TMS Work Takes Time and Psychological Awareness. Physicians in a variety of specialties have a strong science background and are technically skilled, but are often weaker in the psycho-social arena. This includes a lack of training and a lack of interest in emotional factors. On top of this, doctors are often rushed.

Doctors in our health care system are far better paid for doing procedures, injections, surgery, testing, x-rays and MRI scans than they are for counseling a person with pain and listening to and integrating information about their life traumas. This payment system is a major disincentive for many physicians to treat patients with a mind-body approach.

I find the patient stories fascinating. Healing people with a mind-body approach is incredibly rewarding. But minute for minute, it is not lucrative. Patients may not realize that each day my office is open, before a single patient is seen, I have spent $800 to $1,000 on rent, staff salaries, office insurance, staff insurance, worker's compensation, medical malpractice insurance, office supplies, medical supplies, licensing fees and city taxes. There is pressure on many doctors to collect a certain amount of money to cover costs and ensure a decent income. Doing things quickly tends to pay more and mind-body work cannot be rushed.

Every day, I face this push and pull of interests. I am a busy physician with patients who need to see me for a variety of problems, some of them urgent. I am also a mind-body practitioner who wants to spend the necessary time with patients. This allows me to understand their health problems in a detailed fashion and a broader personal context.

With the health care system as it is now, it takes a unique physician who is willing to focus on mind-body work. What might change this? What other factors might contribute to change?

My colleague Dr. Arthur Smith and I have discussed at length the factors that could change the current state of medical practice. He has published a paper on this subject, "HMOs Would Be Wise to Investigate Alternative Ways to Improve Health."(5)

The financial and clinical incentives of the mind-body approach could line up well in a managed care or HMO setting. In this environment, the physicians want to cure people and the business managers want to spend as little money as possible. To include the mind-body approach in the medical group practice would work toward the goal of curing all patients, cost effectively. Our approach still needs to break through the established hierarchy of practitioners, trained in a particular approach or philosophy, who practice evidence-based medicine. This term is widely used, but is often just a synonym for prescribing what drug company-sponsored medication trials select as a more effective pill.

REDUCTIONISM AS THE DOMINANT
MEDICAL PHILOSOPHY

4) Medical doctors, by nature, are mostly reductionist thinkers.

Medical specialties have developed around single organ systems: eye doctor, ear nose and throat, proctology, urology and cardiology, just to name a few.

The problem is that the disciplines have been separated. Not just separated, but these specialists look at a problem with that organ and cannot look beyond it. A person with symptoms gets referred to a specialist for that part of the body. Appropriate evaluation is done and if nothing is found, that specialist is not typically trained in looking farther and wider. Another specialist gets involved and sometimes another.

LOOKING ELSEWHERE FOR A SOLUTION

In my years as a physician, I have found some very serious medical conditions and diagnosed cancer, heart attacks, blood clots and strokes. When symptoms are less specific or last a long time without anyone finding an answer, in this highly technological and sub-specialized era, the answer is usually mind-body.

Some issues to consider:

• Do your symptoms wax and wane or come and go?

• Have doctors not found a clear explanation?

• Is your pain level well above what doctors think you should feel?

• Do physical treatments provide only temporary relief?

• Have doctors put their hands up in confusion, actually or metaphorically, as to why you are suffering so much?

• Do doctors hint or whisper about psychological factors?

• Do you feel better when you are on vacation or distracted?

• Have you had other conditions when you are particularly

stressed, such as TMJ, tension headaches and irritable bowel syndrome?

If you answered "Yes" to any of the above questions, keep reading. I have some answers that may help you.

LOOKING AT SYMPTOMS FOR REAL ANSWERS

You might be asking, "If it is so easy to rule out problems with the body's structure and chemistry, why am I still in pain? Isn't it possible that modern medicine simply isn't able to see what wrong with me?" If that is what you are thinking, you are right. For a vast majority of people, what is causing their pain is not something that shows up on a clinically available scan. It is taking place in the mind/brain.

In this part of the book, you will learn how to see what it is about your mind that might be causing your pain. A questionnaire will help you find the answer.

THE TMS QUESTIONNAIRE

After you have a doctor, or doctors, look you over for physical or structural problems, you might think that you are done. But that is not the case at all.

After ruling out possible but rare structural deficiencies, it is time to look somewhere else for answers. And those answers are likely in your mind. There is not a probe to insert or test that can instantly tell you if you have TMS or not. As is the case in the field of psychology, questionnaires are one of the best ways we have discovered to help patients access their mental state of health on their own.

Below are seven questions I have developed that can give you a good idea if it is your mind/brain that is causing the pain. Answer the questions as accurately as you can and add the total.

I will explain this questionnaire (6) in much more detail in Chapter VIII where I focus on the process of diagnosis.

THE FULL TMS QUESTIONNAIRE

1. Have you noticed a relationship between your pain and your emotional state and stress level just prior to the onset of pain?

Definitely: 2 points

At times: 1 point

Not really: 0 points

2. Would you describe yourself in general as being very hard on yourself, highly responsible for others, very thorough, orderly or a perfectionist?

Definitely: 2 points

I have noticed some of these characteristics: 1 point

Not really: 0 points

3. Have you suffered from other tension-related illnesses such as:

- **hives, eczema, rashes brought on by tension**

- **spastic colon, irritable bowel, gastritis, reflux/heartburn**

- **tension or migraine headaches**

- **unexplained prostate trouble or pelvic pain**

77

• TMJ, teeth grinding, plantar warts

Definitely, two or more categories: 2 points

Yes, at least one: 1 point

No: 0 points

4. Have you been told regarding the cause of your pain that "There's nothing that can be done surgically," "There's nothing wrong," "It's a soft issue problem" or "The cause is degenerative changes"?

Yes: 1 point

No: 0 points

5. Do you spend a fair amount of time during the day thinking and worrying about your pain, researching an answer and obsessing about its cause?

Yes: 1 point

No: 0 points

6. Have you tried several different treatments or approaches for your pain and received only temporary or limited relief from each of them?

Yes: 1 point

No: 0 points

7. Do you find that massage helps your pain significantly or that you are quite sensitive to massage in several parts of your back or neck?

Yes: 1 point

No: 0 points

TOTAL POINTS: _____

Add up all the points for the answers to the questions above and you are on your way to find out if you might be a TMS sufferer. Below is the scoring key, the same one I use when I meet with patients.

If you scored:

7-10 points: Highly probable for TMS

4-6 points: Possible TMS candidate

0-3 points: Probably not a TMS candidate

If you did not score a four or higher, you may wonder if you might have some other condition that is causing you pain. That is why I have developed a few additional questions that might help you see if you might be a borderline TMS case. These questions are:

8. Does the pain ever move to another location in your body or jump around?

_____ Yes _____No

9. Have you noticed the pain improve when you have another tension-related illness?

_____ Yes _____No

10. Has the pain significantly changed or gone away while on vacation, away from home or while distracted?

_____ Yes _____No

If you answered "Yes" to any of the questions above, you might be able to point to TMS as the source of your pain.

Ultimately any diagnosis must be confirmed by a qualified physician.

DISCUSSION

People ask me, "Doesn't everyone score about 6 to 10 points on this? Aren't the questions vague enough that they don't really help to diagnose anyone?"

In my experience, people whom I diagnose and successfully treat with TMS are usually in the 7 to 10 point range with some at 6. On the other hand, I see patients in the office and occasionally some patients download this form from my website, not realizing it is not designed for a blood pressure or knee sprain visit. They typically score 0 to 4 points. While the questionnaire is admittedly a raw tool and one day a more detailed and research-tested one will be available, it has proven to be a helpful guide.

SUB-TYPES OF TMS

What if you took the test and found you have TMS? No, you did not fail. You have started the first step in finding out how to make yourself better. But you might be wondering what is TMS, anyway?

TMS, at its simplest, is a painful condition of muscles and sometimes nerves that is caused by emotional tension, stress and fear of the pain. It is a classic vicious cycle that needs to be broken. The cycle is in the nervous system. The pain is real but it is not a structural disorder.

In a broader sense, TMS is a PPD, a Psycho Physiologic Disorder, a mind-body disorder in which the condition cannot be fully understood without examining the mind/brain and body and cannot be cured without a focus on the role of the central nervous system of brain and emotions. While pain is the most common manifestation, gastrointestinal PPD might cause nausea or diarrhea. Genitourinary PPD might cause urinary frequency or urgency.

TMS comes in several flavors and it can be useful to know where you fall in the spectrum. The key types of TMS are:

• **Pure TMS:** Here, no structural or chemical causes are evident in your body after an examination and appropriate testing by your doctors. There has been no clear explanation prior to TMS and there is nothing structural.

• **TMS with Imaging "Noise":** For example, small disc protrusions in the lumbar spine, which are not impinging on nerves or not compressing the *thecal* sac significantly, are just normal parts of our bodies and not something of concern.

• **Mixed /TMS:** It would be nice if we could all be put into neat compartments, but TMS does not work that way. You might be a prime candidate for TMS regarding personality traits and have a life filled with stressors, all of which aggravate your symptoms. You might also have some evidence of structural issues that bears at least some connection to the pain, such as the shape of your spine causing an impingement of a nerve affecting the side involved.

Surgeons may say that you are not a candidate for surgery, but suggest an epidural, medication or physical therapy to ease the pain. Maybe you have tried all of these temporary solutions, but your pain persists. Many of my patients in this category also noticed that when they are upset or feel strong emotions, their pain worsens and the temporary Band-Aids stop working. You might also be in this category if your symptoms seem out of proportion to findings on imaging. Doctors may notice something on certain x-rays or scans, but your symptoms far exceed in intensity and duration, what would be expected from the imaging results.

This category is the most confusing to patients. They want the 'either/or' response. I have got this, or I do not.

WHEN EITHER/OR IS LESS THAN ENOUGH

One patient wrote to me:

"So this view of TMS does not exactly focus on the pain all being emotional. And relief from pain involves medical as well as mental healing. I guess I am having trouble understanding this since the books I read stressed so much accepting that the cure lies in accepting that nothing physical is wrong and that the pain is caused by emotions. So perhaps another way to look at it is that my pain is caused by emotions and a physical cause. If that is so then I guess I need to do TMS work as well as epidural. I can do that!! Thanks for taking time to answer my questions."

My treatment of each patient is individualized and based upon their history, personality, exam findings and an MRI review. Similarly, my answer for this patient was written to her only:

I responded: "I have a nuanced view of TMS pain that can include ONLY TMS, ONLY STRUCTURAL, or sometimes a combination of the two. It's harder to grab on to, but in your case it is more accurate."

While this represents a relatively small percentage of my overall TMS practice, I think this may be helpful to some of you who struggle with the black and white, either/or approach of some writing in this field.

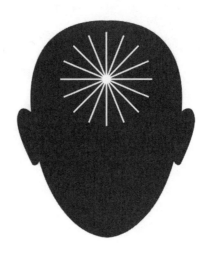

CHAPTER V

Dr. Sarno's Discoveries and Theories Changed Everything

Most fields have their giants. These are the people who show the rest of us a new or better way. Physics has Einstein. Electricity has Thomas Edison. Computing has Steve Jobs. Pain Medicine has Dr. John E. Sarno.

Dr. Sarno challenged the medical establishment to rethink the way it tested for and treated pain. At the same time, he taught patients a new way of thinking about their pain, a diagnostic and treatment model that could lead to relief without medication or surgery.

That is because, as Dr. Sarno described, the problems in many cases were not with the body, but the mind. By meeting and examining tens of thousands of patients over his tenure at the Howard A. Rusk Institute of Rehabilitation Medication at the New York University Medical Center, Sarno had a front-row seat to observe and treat pain. Patients would come to him complaining of crippling pain that did not end.

What Sarno discovered by meeting with countless patients is the equivalent to Thomas Edison's famous experiment to invent the incandescent light bulb. Through hours of time dealing with real-life conditions, not just theory, Edison found a mix of the right material and a vacuum bulb. By talking with countless patients and seeing what worked and what did not, Sarno was the first to create a hypothesis about the exact causes of pain.

Only now, roughly 35 years after Sarno's groundbreaking work, are doctors beginning to be able to peer inside the brain's inner workings and to learn more scientifically what Sarno knew empirically through observation and experience.

This chapter will introduce you to the work of Dr. Sarno. You will see how his experience with real people experiencing real pain helped him to form a way of thinking about pain that we are only now beginning to understand. You will also discover the way the brain can actually create and/or amplify what we experience as physical pain.

MY OWN STORY OF ESCAPING PAIN

Dr. Sarno's genius was taking what he saw in working with patients to figure out something that does not show up in a microscope. It was a classical approach to discovering something about the body, not with test tubes, but by talking to real patients. I should know. I was one of those patients.

I have been a medical doctor for nearly thirty years and have treated thousands of patients who came to me struggling with their chronic pain.

In a way, my pain treatment career started when my own chronic pain was relieved. For three years I had chronic knee pain that I used to think was from a basketball or running injury. After understanding and applying the information that you will be learning in this book, my chronic knee pain became a thing of the past. I did not have to take medicine, do physical therapy or avoid my favorite sports activities.

EARLY INFLUENCES

An early influence of mine was a family doctor who I had during my adolescence. He asked me about stress and tension in relation to my stomach pains. "Are you nervous about parties and social events?"

I also had back spasms triggered by other stressful aspects of being a teenager. My family doctor was not sophisticated in his approach to this mind-body connection in relation to my symptoms. The fact that he gave a voice to the connection proved powerful to me as I got older.

In college, I had severe back spasms two to three times. In retrospect, each appears correlated with emotional stress. I had a hint of that at the time and now I am sure of it. The immediate precipitating factor, playing basketball or squash, might have seemed the most important. In reality, there was more to this pain than met the superficial glance.

MEDICAL SCHOOL STRESSES

In this context I started medical school at New York University (NYU). I found the academic and geographic transition from college to medical school challenging. Medical school involved a lot of intense memorization. College had been more about thinking and understanding concepts, especially in my senior year. To help deal with the new pressures related to medical school, I ran and played basketball.

Eventually, I began to experience knee pain, which became severe enough to considerably limit my participation in my athletic activities. This was discouraging because running and playing basketball were important physical and psychological releases for me.

I embarked on the usual treatments to try to relieve my knee pain, starting with anti-inflammatory medications prescribed by the student health internist. Next, I was sent to an orthopedic specialist who prescribed specific exercises and different anti-inflammatory medicines. My legs became stronger from the exercises, but the pain persisted.

I noticed myself thinking constantly about this problem. Would I play basketball again without pain? Could I resume running along the East River in Manhattan? I was only twenty-one years old and I feared losing the ability to participate in the sports that I loved.

MEETING THE DOCTOR WHO CHANGED EVERYTHING FOR ME

Out of desperation, I sought out a physical medicine and rehabilitation doctor who had lectured to us about several topics in anatomy class. I figured I might be able to get a third opinion or a supervised physical therapy program from him. Instead, I got a life and career-altering response.

Dr. John Sarno looked me in the eye when I described my persistent knee pain and said, "Ninety five percent of chronic pain is psychosomatic. What do you think about that?"

Shocked by his answer, I responded with some comment about migraine headaches and stress, but initially resisted the idea that my chronic knee pain could be stress related. I was an intramural basketball champion from college trying to recapture glory on the basketball courts next to the medical school dorm. What did this have to do with emotions or the mind-body linkage?

Unsurprised by my skeptical response, Dr. Sarno invited me to attend a talk he was giving the following week to a group of his patients. He said that if I were interested, he would then examine me to make a specific diagnosis.

I decided it was worth a try. I was open to psychological, or as he called them, psychosomatic connections and explanations. After all, I was a medical student and intrigued about learning new theories and treatment approaches. Also, I was desperate to seek a cure and willing to try something a little unexpected or unusual to see if it would work.

DR. SARNO'S SEMINAR

My first observation at Dr. Sarno's seminar was surprise at the type of people who attended. They were well-dressed, many were in their 40's and 50's with some in their 30's and 60's. They looked completely healthy on the surface. At 21, I was by far the youngest. In appearance, they were wholly unlike the street people we examined and treated at Bellevue Hospital or the worn-out older men from the Veteran's Administration Hospital next door.

Dr. Sarno shared his ideas with a slide-show presentation. This was back in the 80's before PowerPoint existed. He showed some hand-drawn schematics and some text outline slides. He discussed the history of back pain, which was his focus in the chronic pain area. He wove into this a history and basic explanation of Freudian psychology and the conscious and unconscious mind.

Dr. Sarno then described his own experience treating patients as the Director of Outpatient Rehabilitation at the Rusk Institute and his observations of which patients' chronic pain improved and why. He noted that many of the explanations for people's pain, based upon x-ray findings, were not valid and he cited numerous studies to that effect. (1)

For example, people with scoliosis, the curvature of the spine, or spina bifida occulta, a bony defect at the bottom of the spine, were no more likely to have pain than individuals with normal x-rays. He backed up this observation with published research data that found no correlation between pain and many commonly cited x-ray explanations.

DR. SARNO'S THEORY: TMS

Dr. Sarno went on to detail a mechanism whereby emotional repression, the holding of feelings inside and in the subconscious, would lead the nervous system to send out a fight or flight response, the autonomic nervous system, which could lead to ischemia, the lack of blood flow to muscles and nerves. As a result of this absence of blood flow, painful spasms would be experienced.

Dr. Sarno explained how this process of emotional repression leading to restricted blood flow and then pain was related to certain personality characteristics. He described how the process could be undone by a person becoming aware of and attentive to the feelings, rather than thinking and worrying about the apparent physical causes of the pain.

Others in the audience nodded their heads in acknowledgment or approval, as well. The response from the audience helped convince me I was not alone or crazy in seeing that this made sense. These were people who were educated and experienced and knew when an approach made sense and was not foolishness. Slowly I began to understand this dynamic and decided to apply it to myself.

Dr. Sarno's status as Professor of Rehabilitation Medicine added credibility, along with his white coat, bow tie and assertive manner. Hearing this information from a trained professional who had research to back up his ideas went a long way in helping TMS patients accept the truth of his diagnosis. That same principle holds today.

I did not know what to expect when I went to the seminar, but when it was over two hours later, I left feeling more optimistic and hopeful than I had in quite a while. As I walked home to my small apartment in Manhattan, I thought deeply about the insights and connections that had been made during the talk.

When I got home, I sat down, took off my shoes and reflected on the evening. As I did, I could also feel a weight being removed from my shoulders. The weight was the pressure I was feeling to solve my knee pain dilemma and the worry I was experiencing about it. By the next day I was surprised to notice that I was walking more freely and feeling less pain!

MY CONSULTATION WITH DR. SARNO

Approximately two weeks later, I had a formal consultation with Dr. Sarno who confirmed that I did indeed have the TMS diagnosis with my worrying, perfectionistic personality and the tender points he easily found upon examination of my back.

I followed the program's advice to be more active, to **talk** to my pain and tell it to go away, and to think about my stress at school or with my social life rather than the knee pain itself. Soon I was out jogging a bit and shooting some baskets. I actually resumed full participation in sports over the next month or so without pain.

The experience with Dr. Sarno had a profound impact on me and I wanted to learn as much about his approach as I could. I sought out a summer internship at the Rusk Institute to learn about the field of Rehabilitation Medicine. The following academic year, I continued to share my experiences with my fellow medical students and a few professors, but their skeptical and scoffing responses discouraged me from talking about it too much.

During my second year of medical school, I was able to obtain a work-study research grant and during the following summer, under Dr. Sarno's supervision, I designed and collected data for a research study on the outcomes of treatment for TMS.

The phone interview responses I received from Dr. Sarno's patients were remarkable because a high percentage of patients had similar stories to my own and had been dramatically helped by the mind-body approach. The statistical results that were collected were first reported in Dr. Sarno's book, *Mind Over Back Pain*. (1)

These results and my recovery encouraged me to remain interested and faithful to the promise of the mind-body method as a valid solution for treating pain. Years later, after my residency training was completed and I had begun a small private practice, I reconnected with Dr. Sarno on a visit to New York. He asked, "Do you diagnose TMS?" He then asked, "Are you accepting in referrals?"

My answers were "Yes" and "Yes," but I wondered how many referrals would come from across the continent? To my surprise, Dr. Sarno did receive calls and letters from California and I became his prime referral in the Southern California region.

Although he is now retired from clinical practice, I recently saw a patient who was referred by Dr. Sarno. He is still reading the emails and letters that he receives and continues to honor me by referring Southern California patients to my office.

I am telling you this story to underscore that it is natural to be skeptical about the theory. It is natural to question something that may run so contrary to what other doctors have told you. My skepticism was overcome by my personal experience, by my summer research and, thirty years later, by thousands of successful patients. Now we have to continue to work on yours.

HOW THE MIND/BRAIN CAN CAUSE PHYSICAL PAIN

Our brain is the core of our nervous system. If you have pain, it is because of the brain.

The way it is all connected has to do with the way the body's nerves are built. The best way to think of the body's nervous system is like a river. The main part of the river is the *central nervous system*. The central nervous system is the brain, the spinal cord and the part where all the information about the body's systems is pulled together. Just as a river has branches and tributaries, so too, does our central nervous system.

Branching from the brain and spinal cord are the nerves that comprise our *peripheral nervous system*. The peripheral nervous system spiders its way into every nook and cranny of your body, from your finger tips to the tips of your toes. This peripheral nervous system connects with the central nervous system. Together, these systems form the primary way that our experiences are transmitted to the brain and are interpreted and understood.

How does all this turn into pain? Scientists have very clearly shown what happens in most of these cases. Most pain is acute, fleeting and temporary. A burn, a gust of cold or a pinch affects your body and sets off the peripheral nerves. That negative signal is transmitted to the brain via the spinal cord and we react. Eventually, the pain remits and we go back to our baseline state.

If you have ever touched a hot flame, you just gave your peripheral and central nervous systems a workout. The pain that shot to your spinal cord and brain told you to move away from the heat, not tomorrow, but right now. Sometimes, the painful stimuli persist, such as the prisoner of war who is repeatedly tortured and who cannot get away from the pain and cannot get the pain out of his head.

The difference between forgetting quickly, learning and adapting, versus permanent or long-term effects is the central nervous system's interpretation, understanding and control of the situation or stimulus. A prisoner who has no way to avoid terrible beatings reacts a certain way. Even a dog or cat that is mistreated has a characteristic personality change, tending to shy away from contact, for years or forever.

It is the interpretation that is crucial. The example of the soldier who is shot versus a civilian who is shot in a drive-by illustrates this difference as well. (Chapter I) We believe these differences are found at the *cerebral cortex* and *limbic levels* of the brain, by the kinds of neuronal connections that are made, the memories that are kept in the *hippocampus* and the judgments that continue to be made in the frontal cortex.

The cerebral cortex is the advanced part of the brain that is connected to the body to help us see, hear and experience touch, not to mention handling movement, abstract thought and creativity. The limbic system of the brain is a part of the more primitive brain that handles emotions, memories and behaviors. One such part of the limbic system is the hippocampus, which is focused on allowing us to remember things.

HOW YOUR 'FIGHT OR FLIGHT' TURNS INTO PAIN

Dr. Sarno was one of the first people to start to understand how the brain's messages can result in pain. When you are nervous enough about something, your *autonomic nervous system* kicks in. You may not know the term autonomic nervous system, but you have undoubtedly felt its power. It is your fight-or-flight response. It is the feeling when your hair is standing up on the back of your neck as you walk into a dark alley and you see something move. Suddenly, all your senses go into hyper drive. Even the quiet shuffling of your shoes on the ground sounds like a giant earthmover, because your brain is turning up the volume.

Sometimes the autonomic nervous system can be a huge help. If there is a bad guy lurking in the corner with a lead pipe, the autonomic system gives you Spiderman-like hearing. You will know about the threat and your brain can get your muscles ready to fight or your legs prepared to sprint. The example of the mother lifting a car off her child is another benefit of the adrenalin secreted in the fight or flight response.

The problem is that this same fight or flight response can get triggered when situations are not necessarily life-or-death. This problem is what causes pain when the body is fine. Dr. Sarno first hypothesized the autonomic nervous system produced changes in blood flow via the peripheral nervous system and that these changes led to painful areas in the neck, back and elsewhere. The mechanism still is not totally clear, even 35 years later.

However, examples abound when a person is worrying about something. This worry and anxiety puts the brain's limbic system into hyper drive. This excitability of the limbic system then puts the body in its fight-or-flight mode, even though the person might be sitting in a quiet office, not in a dark alley. When you keep this fight-or-flight mode activated long enough, the person might experience pains in the chest, stomach or back.

Interestingly, though, when the worry abates, the pain vanishes. When the worry goes away, the central nervous system stops sending signals and stops amplifying otherwise normal sensory input from the peripheral nervous system. In this case, when the negative emotion goes away, the pain goes away.

THE 'IMPRINTING OF PAIN'

The fight-or-flight system is a great way to understand just how emotions can create pain. But it is not the only way this can work. Another way emotions create pain is with the so-called imprinting of pain. This pain may start with an injury, something that would ordinarily resolve itself, such as a bumped knee, a pulled muscle or a strained back. However, as you think about the pain more and more and it becomes a near obsession, the nervous system starts to hang onto the pain sensation. By repeatedly thinking about the pain and "babying your bad back," you are teaching your brain that there is a problem. Repetition is practice. If you practiced the piano every day, your fingers would learn to dance over the keys. So it goes with pain. Repetition is repeating an experience such as a feeling from your body or a thought, which causes neurons to grow and solidify. By "practicing your pain," chemical changes in your body occur to make that pathway more powerful and more significant. The focus on pain reinforces the pain.

Again, think of the beginning piano player trying to strike the keys properly and the expert who effortlessly moves his fingers, from thought to playing, the intermediate steps are made routine and the pathways solidified.

Pain is like this when it persists. The pathways become more firmly embedded, the transmission stronger and the input gets amplified. On top of this, the central nervous system's response to the signals is increased attention and increased focus.

THE WONDERS OF MODERN BRAIN IMAGING

Thanks to the advances in imaging technologies, we can look inside the body and see how this works.

When you stick your head in an MRI machine, doctors can see what portions of your brain are activated or "lit up." When patients with long-standing pain are examined, what we see is staggering. **What we now know is that people with chronic pain often have the emotional portions of their brains lit up.**

This part of our brain controls a number of functions, including blood flow. The more you think about the pain, the more attention your brain pays to it. Focus and attention amplifies the experience of pain and distracts the central nervous system from other important tasks, such as moving, talking or feeling.

Again, this should not come as a total surprise. Where our attention goes, so goes our brainpower. Think of the driving advice you got from your first instructor, "Keep your eyes moving and aim high in steering." If you stare at something, you steer toward it. If you stop looking at it and keep moving your eyes, it is easier to keep balance.

It is true the stress, the worry, the fear and the anger impinge us from the outside. But these feelings also affect us on the inside. Our brains are literally rewired to focus on the pain, not on the rest of our surroundings. We can see these changes in the functional MRI imaging of chronic pain. Pain replaces the sound of babbling brooks and the giggles of our children. It is a process of growing the wrong connections, building the wrong neural pathways and amplifying the wrong signals. It is a cycle out of control, a vicious feedback loop toward pain and toward failure.

BREAKING THE VICIOUS CYCLE

How do you get out of this debilitating cycle? This is the

transformation that is the promise of this book. The transformation is from someone who is miserable, in pain, worried, fearful and hopeless to someone who has a future, has a life, has hope and can take action. The brain pain transformation program is what it sounds like. It starts at the central nervous system, the cortex, the thinking brain and the thoughts. This shift in attention at the anterior cingulate and pre-frontal cortex causes a reversal of the process that got you in trouble in the first place.

It is important to note that while the transformation short-circuits these counterproductive pathways, it does not eliminate them completely. The nervous system seems to retain them at some level as evidenced by the many people who years later have a 'shadow' or 'echo' pain in the same area of their body. The peripheral nervous system, triggered by some memory or some emotional experience, can bring these negative feelings back. With knowledge, you will know how to keep these episodes brief.

SARNO AND FREUD

Certainly Dr. Sarno's writings are imbued with Sigmund Freud's theories and perspectives. Dr. Sarno clearly shows Freud a great deal of respect for his own seminal insights into human psychology. The models of repression and unconscious feelings, such as anger, rage and fear, derive from this body of knowledge.

Contemporary psychology and psychologists, along with psychiatrists and many physicians, at least those who care, have moved very far from the Freudian perspective in Dr. Sarno's books and this is one of the criticisms, stated or implied, of his work.

In addition to successfully treating patients with psychophysiological disorders such as TMS, my goal has been to find ways to bridge the gap between Sarno's seminal contributions and modern medicine. A good place to start is to see whether biologic descriptions of the brain integrate with Freud's theories.

An excellent review of this was written by Mark Solms and published in May 2004. (2) Some of the points made in this piece describe the roots of psychology:

• Freud's explanations of the mind dominated the first half of the 1900's.

• The basic proposition was that motivations remain hidden in the unconscious mind.

• Repressive forces withhold them from consciousness.

• The ego, the executive apparatus of the mind, rejects the motivations.

• The unconscious drives the id, prompting behavior that is unacceptable or uncivilized.

• Repression is necessary as the drives express unconstrained passions, fantasies, aggression or sexual urges.

• Mental illness is when repression fails.

• The aim of psychotherapy is to trace symptoms back to the unconscious roots and expose them to mature rational thought, depriving them of power.

This was based upon observation, not controlled experimentation.

During the second half of the 1900's, the use of new medications gained ground and biological approaches overshadowed analysis.

INTEGRATING FREUD AND FUNCTIONAL MRI

Can all of this be integrated? Biology, medications, fMRI and Freud's theories? Some very well-known people are trying to do this, such as the International Neuro-Psychoanalysis Society, Nobel laureate Eric Kandel, A. Damasio, Panksepp, Schacter and Wolf Singer. (3)

Today's findings confirm the existence and role of unconscious mental processing. An example is the different memory systems of the explicit (conscious) and the implicit (unconscious). In 1996, LeDoux demonstrated a pathway under the cortex (thinking/conscious) that connects perceptual information with primitive brain structures (where fear is experienced). This bypasses the hippocampus (conscious memories) and hence current events can trigger emotionally important past events, including irrational fears (e.g. "bearded men worry me"). (4)

Another finding is that the brain structures for explicit memory are not formed during the first two years of life (hence what Freud called infantile amnesia). We cannot recall these memories to consciousness, but that does not mean they cannot affect adult feelings and behavior. (2)

Is repression a reality? Patients with brain damage to the right parietal region are unaware of certain physical defects, but with brain stimulation may notice these post-stroke problems. Once stimulation was turned off, the patient reverted to her prior belief that nothing was wrong **and** forgot the part of the interview where she had acknowledged her problem! Ramachandran therefore concluded that memories can be selectively repressed. (5)

Patients with damage to the inhibitory structures of the brain, the frontal limbic region, do in fact release irrational thoughts when questioned by therapists or researchers. The thoughts are not random, but do appear to recast reality as the patient wishes it to be. Is this "Freud's pleasure principle?" (2)

With regard to the id, neuroscientists compare our brains to those of lower animals and find remarkable similarities.

Modern neuroscientists, however, do not accept the dichotomy between sexuality and aggressive instincts. They focus on 'reward', 'anger and rage', 'fear and anxiety' and 'panic' systems. This broadening is consistent with my belief that emotions such as fear and panic do play a significant role and in some people replace the anger and rage root described in the works of Sarno and Freud.

The seeking system resembles the libido, a pleasure seeking system. Research implicates this system in craving and addiction. Recent work on dreams indicates that the seeking system may also play a role in dreams. This has replaced data suggesting that dreams are purely related to brainstem chemical changes that had nothing to do with emotion or motivation.

Perhaps this is 'retrofitting' of new data. Perhaps it is wishful thinking, but I believe that Freud, a neurologist interested in pharmacology and science himself, would be pleased at the science available now to study the mind/brain.

In subsequent chapters, I will come back to both research evidence and clinical approaches to try to explain this powerful phenomenon of emotions linked to pain.

CHAPTER VI

Understanding Pain with Relevant Scientific Evidence

What exactly is the evidence that the diagnosis, theory, approach, which has been referenced and briefly discussed, and the understanding that underlies the rest of this book, is true?

Unfortunately, at this time, we lack the multi-million dollar government or pharmaceutical funding that could provide the "knock your socks off" scientific evidence. In the mind/body field, we also work in a realm of medicine less conducive to the research comparing the effects of a yellow active pill versus the yellow inert pill. "Evidence based medicine" forms a lot of the evidence for one type of chemotherapy versus another. Or one blood pressure pill versus another.

SIX TYPES OF EVIDENCE

1) The experiences of tens of thousands of patients treated by the coterie of TMS doctors.

2) The experiences of these same physicians, including many who have been treated or self-treated successfully themselves.

3) A small number of published research studies, admittedly none a definitive controlled, double-blind study.

4) Research conducted on the brain and on patients with pain

or emotional issues that supports the mechanisms and approaches discussed here.

5) Functional MRI (fMRI) data, while not specifically done to test TMS, supports its premises and conclusions.

6) The lack of success of many conventional approaches, not to mention the high cost of same.

Regarding Point 1, you can read this book and other TMS books by Drs. Sarno, Sopher, Selfridge, Schubiner, Hanscom and others to hear anecdotal testimonials. (See References and Resources sections.)

These and other physicians and psychotherapists describe Point 2 again in books and websites.

Regarding Point 3, a list of these references and more discussion of the studies I have published are in this book's Research Chapter (Chapter XI) and also in Appendix: References.

Here is a discussion about Points 4 and 5:

For many years, physicians have known that physical pain and depression are intertwined. (1) In fact, up to 80% of patients with depression have mainly physical symptoms. (2) Doctors have treated pain with antidepressants, such as tricyclic medications, for years as well. Shown in a study for patients with chronic tension headaches, these medications, along with relaxation strategies, combined for better results than either alone. (3) This is fairly generic knowledge, but it does show that the mind-body link in pain has been approached from other viewpoints.

Another connection is that the neurotransmitters serotonin and norepinephrine are involved in the regulation of external and internal sensation. These are the chemicals that transmit information and feeling in the brain, that are altered by anti-depressant medications and presumably by depression itself. This is what I mean when I state that the brain is constantly modifying and responding to sensations from the body via the spinal cord, ignoring some and amplifying others, such as chronic pain. In depressed people, these sensations are not usually ignored and may be experienced as more uncomfortable or even painful. (4)

fMRI RESEARCH STUDIES

Regarding Point 5, modern imaging technology used on the brain is a key tool in proving this, up-until-now, nebulous connection between mind and body. It is interesting because imaging of the body has some value, but imaging of the brain and indirectly the mind might be where the true answers lie. A method of imaging you will read about here is fMRI or functional MRI scanning. Unlike regular MRI's that show three dimensional images of the scanned region (the structures), functional MRI's focus on the function in that region.

One aspect of function commonly measured is blood flow. Logically, the more blood flow to an area of the brain means that this area is being used. It is like looking at a building, where the power is on and being used, when the people are working.

Such studies have shown that the brain "parallel processes" emotional and physical pain. UCLA researchers, Drs. Eisenberger and Lieberman, have shown that social rejection lights up the brain regions in fMRI studies. This is important in the response to physical pain at the Dorsal Anterior Cingulate Cortex. (5) Social rejection is an emotional experience and physical pain is a "physical experience." Yet in the brain there are very similar patterns of activity. This implies that physical pain and social rejection "hurt" in the same way. This relates to our ongoing point that what you feel and what you think greatly affects, and we believe can cause, your pain problem.

Dr. Lieberman from UCLA calls the anterior cingulate cortex the "neural alarm system." From there, signals proceed to higher regions that act to deal with the pain. The right ventral pre-frontal cortex (RVPFC) helps dampen the emotional distress caused by pain. (5) Perhaps the program described later in this book and the work we do to change people's perception of pain and reduce their fear enhances the dampening of the RVPFC.

A fascinating study by Derbyshire looked at pain generated from hypnotic suggestion. This experience of pain felt very real to the subjects. On the fMRI, changes were seen within the thalamus, Anterior cingulate (ACC), insula and prefrontal and parietal cortices. These findings "compare well with the activation patterns during pain from nociceptive (physical pain) sources" and provide the "first direct experimental evidence in humans linking specific neural activity with the immediate generation of a pain experience." (6) The authors go on to comment: "The known interconnection of stress, negative affect and pain, inputs from higher neural centers, can expand, amplify or **create** pain symptoms. Taken together, these hypotheses and data raise the possibility that an experience of pain can originate exclusively within a subject's brain or mind rather than being necessarily dependent on the pathology of peripheral tissue."

This is truly a remarkable finding and conclusion that lends powerful neuro-imaging support to the TMS model/hypothesis. The pain is truly "in the brain." This study appears to confirm the idea that pain can originate in the brain and does not require a physical injury to originate!

On his blog, Dr. Ken Pope discussed the details of a study by Dr. Kong, published in the Journal Pain. (7) fMRI scanning was used to try to identify the loci of pain modulation by non-pharmacologic approaches. Dr. Kong wrote, "The experience of pain can be significantly influenced by expectancy (predictive cues). This ability to modulate pain has the potential to affect therapeutic analgesia substantially and constitutes a foundation for non-pharmacological pain relief... Functional magnetic resonance imaging results suggested that brain regions pertaining to the frontoparietal network (prefrontal and parietal cortex) and a pain/emotion modulatory region (rostral anterior cingulate cortex) are involved in cue modulation..."

CHRONIC PAIN LINKED TO EMOTIONAL CENTERS

How does pain go from acute to chronic and why does that matter? Acute pain usually goes away. Back pain studies have shown that 50% of patients are healed in a week or two. 90% heal in eight weeks. (8) What explains the persistence of back pain? For a small percentage of people there is a structural issue that needs to be addressed. Some of these folks suffered major trauma to precipitate the event.

For a significant percentage of pain that persists, however, it is the brain and nervous system that changes, not the back! fMRI studies were compared on people with recent low back pain to those with one to ten years of pain. (9) These researchers found a shift in brain functioning in people with chronic pain of more than one year. In the acute phase, portions of the brain focused on pain and reward are dominant. As pain becomes chronic, the activity of the circuits, which are emotion-based (amygdala and basal ganglia, medial prefrontal cortex), grows in strength. This persists even for people with ten years of pain.

The authors note that the perception of pain is different when experienced through the pain and reward circuits versus the emotion and reward circuits later on. This brain circuit shift occurs over a year and then remains stable. Patients with ten years of pain demonstrate the same brain functional changes. They also comment that the persistence of the condition orients the subject toward suffering.

This clearly and powerfully supports our work and demonstrates that moving the chronic pain patient from the emotional, fearful state they often present towards a more positive, action-oriented style is crucial. This shift leads to a change in regards to the neural circuits and pathways within the brain—away from those troubling emotional brain circuits back towards the conscious and cognitive brain centers. In addition, our treatment program helps the patient to acknowledge and release/express emotions, perhaps disconnecting these emotional circuits in which the pain is enmeshed.

This study falls into the literature on chronification. These are papers where researchers, doctors and psychologists attempt to explain why some patients develop chronic pain, while others do not. It is clear to me that better, more empathetic and clearer diagnosis and treatment early on, can help prevent chronic pain. Emotionally vulnerable individuals should have extra help during those first few months to help prevent ongoing symptoms. Finally, understanding these chronic brain changes helps to confirm why we have the success we do in our program of mind-body healing.

ATTENTION, DISTRACTION AND PAIN

Although this study just touches upon an artificial type of pain and a structured type of distraction, it is interesting because we get a window into brain function with and without distraction. Painful thermal stimuli were used (Ouch!) and a cognitive distraction technique was utilized. Bantick and colleagues concluded, "When subjects were distracted during painful stimulation, brain areas associated with the affective division of the anterior cingulate cortex (ACC) and orbitofrontal regions showed increased activation. In contrast, many areas of the pain matrix (i.e. thalamus, insula, cognitive division of the ACC) displayed reduced activation, supporting the behavioral results of reduced pain perception."(9)

We can certainly speculate that the relief many patients feel with distraction, in benign but painful TMS conditions, may also involve a shift in attention and a shift in brain blood flow and focus, as well.

CONVENTIONALISTS WHO QUESTION
THE ORTHODOXY

Researchers have argued that back pain can be a "surrogate complaint" and often not the primary reason for a visit to the doctor.

Nortin Hadler, M.D., an academic Rheumatologist wrote, "Patients say, "My back hurts but... I'm really here because I can't cope with this episode right now." (10)

To take this a step farther, the back hurts, but the patient cannot cope with life right now and that is why they are in the doctor's office. But will the doctor ask, "What's going on in your life?" Will the doctor be comfortable with a follow-up on this as well? At this time, that prospect is more unlikely than likely.

"I have come to believe that 80% of the experience of chronic pain is emotional," wrote Dr. Mel Pohl, a clinical assistant professor of the Department of Psychiatry and Behavioral Sciences at the Nevada School of Medicine. (11)

J. Coste and associates demonstrated that many of the subjects in their study reported lower quality of life (QOL) in the month prior to the back pain episode and prior to the office visit. (12) As one's quality of life deteriorates, emotional life is uneven, unstable or depressing and the back is affected. That is the conclusion I draw from this reported relationship between QOL and back pain episodes.

CHILDHOOD STRESS AND PAIN

What about research on childhood and young adulthood? Is there support for a connection between emotions in these years and later physical health?

A study done in London suggests that stress in your 20's may lead to low back pain in your 30's. (13) In fact, individuals interviewed at age 23 who reported psychological distress were two and one half times more likely to report having low back pain at age 33.

Researchers in Brazil found that children with back pain were more likely to have hyperactivity and emotional symptoms than matched controls. (14)

Another study looking at people with functional gastrointestinal (GI) disorders, such as irritable bowel and heartburn, found that childhood "adversity," especially in severe form, is an independent predictor for later GI symptoms. (15) There is a close association, in my experience and those of other doctors, between a diagnosis of irritable bowel syndrome and TMS.

Schofferman and colleagues published a study in 1992 that childhood trauma correlated with unsuccessful lumbar spine surgery. (16)

POINT 4, TREATMENT RESEARCH

I find it fascinating when research done for different purposes connects with the work I do with patients. Moseley of Australia has published extensively, and in one study, demonstrated the benefit of "reconceptualization of the problem" after pain physiology education. He took a patient with chronic low back pain and performed fMRI scans prior to and after 2.5 hours of one-to-one teaching about the nervous system and the pain system. He used pictures, examples and metaphors, as we do. A final scan was done and there was a marked reduction in cortical activation. This did not involve the so-called pain matrix, which he defines as the cingulate, frontal or insular cortices. Simply put, education changed the way the brain responded to a physical activity (abdominal contractions). (17)

Bell and Meadows did a study for children with recurrent abdominal pain. It was a brief intervention, a "single one-hour session including psycho-education and coaching of breathing retraining." Pain improved. The treatment was TMS-like or TMS-lite. (18)

Von Korff and Associates had an interesting observation in a paper they wrote and published in the Journal Spine in 2005. (19) He wrote, "More than 80% of individuals with chronic spinal pain have other chronic diseases and pain syndrome." He worried that doctors are treating each complaint as a new condition when these patients have a chronic and more global problem.

He and his colleagues noted that chronic back pain has a substantial overlap with widespread pain and/or fibromyalgia. "About a third of low back pain sufferers at any given time will have widespread pain," Croft said. (20)

These comments and observations are consistent with the TMS model. For one, these patients are often misdiagnosed and treated, symptom focused rather than root cause (nervous system, mind/brain) focused. Furthermore his observation of the "Whack a Doodle" game (hit the object somewhere, it pops up somewhere else) is what we call, I believe more eloquently, "symptom migration" or symptom substitution. TMS symptoms can move from one area of the body to another when incompletely addressed or treated. (Chapter X) Furthermore, he is right again that most of these patients do not just have a localized pain issue, but a more diffuse one. In our conceptualization, this is a chronic nervous system issue, not an acute condition.

Stanford Psychiatrist Dr. F. Maeda and colleagues (21) began to test subjects who were given feedback on their brain's response to painful stimuli and could learn to reduce the pain by roughly 25% after a brief period of training. This change in "thinking" causing pain relief is something that Sarno taught us over 35 years ago and that my patients have been doing for over 25 years with great success. Doctor Maeda used powerful and expensive equipment to connect patients to their "physiology." I believe we teach people to develop this awareness in a more low-tech, less expensive, but highly effective manner.

There is a lot of research on the power of journaling for relief of physical symptoms. (See Chapter IX.) In 1999, J. M. Smyth and associates published a paper with a descriptive title, "Effects of Writing about Stressful Experiences on Symptom Reduction in Patients with Asthma or Rheumatoid Arthritis: A Randomized Trial." (22) The title captures the essence, but simply put, writing expressively and writing about feelings was shown to be far more effective for these two conditions than writing about a person's plans for the day. Note that

RA is an inflammatory condition and asthma also has a significant inflammatory component.

Inflammation is heavily influenced by the immune system. RA can be quite painful. Both conditions improved, 47% had clinically relevant improvement, in the expressive writing group. Improvement was not only subjective, but also featured improvement in lung function measurements and disease activity in RA. This study and others support the idea that writing expressively, or journaling as I call it, can be clinically effective. Perhaps we need the pen and paper companies to send out representatives to doctors' offices to compete with the pharmaceutical representatives?!

PERFECTIONISM AND ITS DANGERS

Clinical research, some of it from Canada, on the effects of perfectionism (one of the Type T personality characteristics discussed in Chapter III) finds a higher risk for irritable bowel syndrome (a mind-body disorder), insomnia, post-partum depression and other health issues. (23) (24) Coping with these conditions and symptom levels were found to be amplified in individuals who scored high on a perfectionist questionnaire.

FEAR OF PAIN IN CHRONIC PAIN

Turk and Wilson published a paper reviewing evidence on chronic pain. (25) They specifically emphasized the "fear of pain" and activity, driven by the "anticipation of pain and increased injury" that reinforces avoidance behavior and keeps people more disabled and paradoxically in more pain.

Fear of movement has a medical name "kinesiophobia." I see this in patients that I examine with chronic pain, especially of the back. I believe that one of the ways we succeed with TMS treatment is getting people to stop being afraid, to understand that pain is NOT damage (Lesson 4) and to start moving again.

Even for those not as psychologically minded, if one helps them break through the fear of the painful condition, they may progress rapidly on a positive, rather than a vicious, cycle.

Patient Example:

I saw this patient recently:

A man in his forties, fairly successful, had pain in his groin area for five years. The pain started in the penile region and he saw specialists who gave him a diagnosis of a hernia, then prostatitis. After hernia repair, however, the pain was severe and continued.

When I saw him, his recent three month pain was perineal, in the area between his testis and anus. At times the pain was excruciating. He had seen a urologist and was treated for prostatitis. After his prostate exam, the pain seemed to shift or move from more in the penile area to the perineum. He reported having prostate pain on and off since the age of 13. The pain was very severe after hernia repair.

His recent psycho-social life included a new supervisory job and an extra-marital friendship that developed into something more.

This patient has also had hip pain, labrum tears in the hip and pinching pains in that area. Yoga helped and then he developed *piriformis* and back issues. He tried physical therapy for years without major improvement. He learned of TMS through reading a book a few months before; the book felt like it applied to him. He tried to wean himself off muscle relaxants and accomplished that task within a few weeks. When the perineal pain improved, it seemed to move around.

Questioning him further, I learned he was a Type T personality. He is the first born in his family, a high achiever and usually very responsible. At age 17, his father was murdered. He had early success in college but feels like his father's death slowed him financially and limited his college choices. Also, his career had not headed in the direction that he had hoped. His current job paid well but was not fulfilling. Married to his beautiful high school sweetheart, he remained curious about other women and felt guilty about this as well. He had two children.

On examination, he had tender points in the left more than the right trapezius muscle and left quadratus lumborum, bilateral IT band and right gluteal. An MRI review showed a bulging disc L4-5 with no nerve impingement, which was otherwise fine.

My diagnosis was TMS. I counseled him about the mind-body connection in chronic pain, the Twelve Stages of Healing and specific examples of shifting his thinking from physical to psychological and away from structural concerns. (See Chapter X.) He obtained the Home Educational Program and was given a referral for a TMS therapist.

The First Follow-Up Visit

He returned several weeks later, noticing improvement. The pain in his perineal region was no longer constant, now intermittent. He no longer needed a cushion or pad while sitting at work. His left hip was no longer causing him much pain and he felt more strength there. He found two therapy sessions to be helpful and intended to continue.

He reported, "The workbook was very helpful," and he listened to the audio CDs. He had begun to often see a connection, but not always, between pain and its emotional triggers.

The Second Follow-Up Visit

The patient returned about a month later.

He had noticed more improvement since his last visit. He was now having more days without perineal pain and occasional days with pain. A rare stiffness in his left hip appeared; he was usually able to attribute the pain to a stressful situation. The workbook was now completed and it had been very helpful to him.

Now the main area of pain is in his foot or plantar fascia. Since his first visit with me, he has improved 80%. At this visit, I emphasized the concept that "pain does not equal damage," helping him to fully accept and confirm that this method is working. I wanted to strengthen his belief in the diagnosis and the approach.

The Third Follow Up Visit

About a month later, his pain was almost gone. He was feeling the pain 3% of the time. The patient was told that he had a stress fracture in his foot by a podiatrist and was put in a walking boot. He had been riding his bicycle more, even prior to the fracture diagnosis, and he was feeling more optimistic.

I will see him back again and perhaps help him with the "stress fracture" diagnosis, as it was not clear to me regarding his mechanism of injury. He has been running more and also biking a lot. He is a TMS success. He is going to work on the final 3% with the home program and his TMS therapist for now.

XRAY FINDINGS ARE OFTEN MISLEADING

Dr. Sarno does a great job refuting the simplicity of the structural model and treatment approach, especially for chronic back pain. He cites many studies that demonstrate that x-ray findings are often misleading, while the general public, chiropractors and some medical doctors often use the x-ray to diagnose and define a patient's back pain. Scoliosis, degenerative changes and wear and tear are rarely the cause of pain.

OSTEOARTHRITIS IN THE SPINE HAS
LITTLE SIGNIFICANCE

Dr. Schneider's research shows that spinal osteoarthritis has little functional significance. (26) Schneider and colleagues at UCSD examined the spines of men and women living in California. These subjects were 60 to 98 years old. Specifically they looked at bone density through DEXA (bone density) testing. An independent radiologist assessed the amount of arthritis and osteoporosis, where the bone softens or thins. Significant spinal osteoarthritis was evident in approximately 40% of these individuals. Arthritis, not surprisingly, increased steadily with age. However, older men with osteoarthritis almost never reported limitations in daily activities. Among older women, about 15% had problems in bending and about 11% had trouble getting out of cars. However, they also experienced few limitations in walking, housework and daily living.

This study is consistent with many other studies showing that wear and tear (osteoarthritis or degenerative changes) progresses as we get older, but usually does not lead to functional concerns. Similarly, wear and tear worsens as we get older, but the peak of back and neck pain, as a significant, disabling issue, is far younger, in the 40's and 50's, surprisingly not the 70's and 80's.

DEGENERATIVE CHANGES ARE OF
LITTLE IMPORTANCE

Correlate this fascinating study with the Boden study, (27) which found that 93% of subjects, aged 60-80, had degenerative changes on an MRI at one or more spinal levels. The vast majority of these had no pain and no interference with function.

If you have degenerative or osteoarthritic changes on x-rays, think of them as 'gray hair of the spine', aging changes of no significance.

JENSEN STUDY OF DISCS IN PEOPLE WITHOUT SYMPTOMS

If you are younger, note that the classic Jensen Study from the New England Journal of Medicine, (28) scanned 98 asymptomatic people, ages 20 through 80, with an average age of 42. Many people without back pain had disc bulges and protrusions. In fact 52% of the subjects had a bulge of at least at one level. 27% had a protrusion. 38% had more than one abnormality. Again, these were people without pain. Therefore, the presence of an MRI finding must be carefully evaluated, as many are of no significance at all.

THE RELATIONSHIP BETWEEN NEW MRI FINDINGS AND SERIOUS LOW BACK PAIN

Dr. Eugene Carragee and his team at Stanford published a paper in The Spine Journal in 2006, which won the "Outstanding Paper Award." (29) Their study included 200 subjects and patients who were followed for five years and had baseline MRI scans. Every six months, there was a telephone interview. New MRI scans were done within 6 to 12 weeks at the start of an episode of new low back pain and compared to baseline images that had no symptoms.

They concluded that over the five years, 51 people had painful low back episodes. Only three had pain, primarily down the leg. Of the 51 patients, 84% had an MRI that was unchanged or had shown improvement! The most common progressive findings were disc signal loss (10%), facet arthrosis (10%) or end plate changes (4%). Only two patients had new findings of "probable clinical significance" and both had primarily leg pain.

What did they notice about these 51 patients, 25% of the total group? They were more likely to have baseline psychological distress (!) and previously disputed worker's compensation claims. New findings were not more frequent in subjects whose episodes began after minor trauma, like a fall, than spontaneously.

They concluded that **most new changes represent progressive age changes not associated with acute events.** This excellent study really de-emphasizes the power and significance of the MRI test in pain and also does a great job following people over time. The minor changes that occur with age are of no significance.

CHAPTER VII

Instructive Patient Stories

These healing stories show the symptoms that people have and the process they go through to get better.

This chapter focuses on case examples. As in all examples in this book, they are based upon real people, but the ages, genders and occupations have been jumbled up to preserve anonymity. Their names have of course been changed.

RICH'S STORY

A 35-year-old man came to the office recently. He had pain for over three years after an accident. The accident was not a minor one. In the weeks after the accident, the immediate pain was not terrible. The accident could have been a lot worse. It was sort of like falling over the handlebars of your bike, landing on your head and having a concussion, but not breaking your neck or back. The initial doctors did x-rays and reassured him that he would heal. His concussion improved, but his neck and lower back pain gradually became worse.

He also related to me that his mother, who was ill with cancer, died about four months after his accident. The final days with her were difficult, but rewarding. His pain continued and even worsened. During this time, he was moving his career forward, with ups and downs, but generally he was on an uphill path to success. His neck and back continued to hurt. He finally got MRI scans of both areas. The lumbar spine was completely normal. The cervical (neck) spine showed a minor bulge, about as small as one can measure and nothing of any significance to explain his pain.

As I spoke with him, it was clear he understood that he was one of those folks who are extremely hard on themselves. A 10/10 on the Type T scale. It was something he was working on and he was in a supportive relationship. He had spent some time previously working out some issues from childhood. There were some financial conflicts in the family, as well, but he was working to solve these.

When I examined him, I was initially impressed that he appeared fit, despite three years that he described as relatively inactive. He was able to bend forward and touch his palms to the floor. His range of motion was normal or above normal in all regards of the neck and back. His neurological examination was also completely normal. I checked reflexes, sensory response and muscle strength: totally intact and fine. I next examined him for the tender points characteristic of TMS. Dr. Sarno first described six of these and this patient was tender in four of the six. (See Chapter VIII.) When I examined his spine, it was completely non-tender, but the muscles adjacent to his spine, in the neck, upper back and lower back, the quadratus lumborum and longissimus, were taut to my examination. He had spasm evident in these muscles.

I diagnosed him as TMS. 100% TMS. Now why do muscles go into spasm? Muscles respond to nerves, which control their contraction and relaxation. Muscles are sent into spasm in response to a trigger such as pure stress, injury plus stress and injury; this is a protective phenomenon. This protection is to guard the area that was hurt, or perceived as hurt. This guarding, physiologically, should last a few days and then gradually release. Exceptions might be an untreated fracture or some other rare, serious condition.

So why might "protective" spasms continue in this patient or individuals like him? Anxiety and fear. Fear that he had a severe injury. Anxiety that he might have died. Worry about his ill parent. Stress in his life. His personality was a Type T. The spasm had basically persisted for three years by the time I saw him. He felt temporarily better during a massage, where the muscles are stretched, kneaded and prodded. But this myofascial pain had lasted far beyond its need or its benefit to the patient. This was how TMS manifested in this gentleman. This is why purely physical treatments had not succeeded. The stress kept the autonomic nervous system, the fight or flight response, very aroused. Hence, the muscles were taut as if ready to explode in an instant.

My plan for him was:

a) Counseling in the office about the diagnosis and prognosis.

b) Discussion of the Twelve Stages of Healing. (Chapter X)

c) Discussion of the concept that pain does NOT mean damage. (Lesson Four)

d) Home program (book, CD, DVD, workbook and journaling)

I told him I expected him to do well. Based upon prior patients with similar symptoms, findings and personality, his prognosis was excellent.

What made him an especially likely success with my TMS healing program?

1) He was open, a little desperate and insightful about his personality.

2) He had a normal MRI. He was certainly reassured by my review, along with his very benign physical examination with a great range of motion.

3) He had no other treatments or diagnoses currently competing for his attention. I felt he would devote himself to this program and this diagnosis.

4) Because he was a former athlete, I felt that he probably had a good pain tolerance. Once he started becoming more active, he would overcome the currently self-imposed limitations on exercise, sports and daily living.

JEFF'S STORY

Here is another patient who illustrates various aspects of the symptoms and recovery from TMS. Let us call him Jeff. When I first met him more than seven years ago, Jeff was a married man in his early 40's, with young children. He was a successful corporate businessman. He was, however, anxious and specifically very worried about his health. His primary symptom was back and calf pain.

He told me that he had a colonoscopy and was told it was fine. The next day, his middle back started to hurt. Subsequently he began to have calf pain and saw a doctor who told him, "This could be serious." This opinion scared him a lot. By the time I saw Jeff, he had seen a couple of physical therapists and a chiropractor. He had not improved.

I talked to him and there was stress with his work, stress with his young children, issues with his wife and a lot of fear of his pain. He was worried and he was anxious. This is understandable with back pain. Fear is part of the problem and part of the solution. We talked quite a bit about his childhood, his family life and his work. He seemed more comfortable as he shared some important details with me.

His orthopedic and neurological exam was normal. Jeff was hesitant to move his back and he did have five out of the six tender points. I reviewed x-rays and MRI scans and found nothing of significant concern. Just some "gray hair" of the spine, so to speak, a little wear and tear many of us get by our 40's. Sometimes this occurs earlier, sometimes later, just like gray hair.

We talked about TMS. Jeff was interested in proceeding in the healing curriculum. In addition to the home program and office advice, I felt he would benefit from seeing a therapist. He did not live close enough to see one of the TMS psychotherapy specialists in my area, face to face. This was before SKYPE. Jeff did do telephone therapy for a while with one of our local therapists and also found an insightful general therapist in his area.

120

His course was not an overnight cure. He did improve, but then he got worse again. There was very much a waxing and waning course of his pain. Jeff gradually learned to connect his pain with his emotional state and issues, but a lot of anxiety interfered with his full acceptance of the diagnosis and recovery.

Jeff kept working at it because overall he felt better than he had before the TMS diagnosis and mind-body healing program. I was able to see him sporadically, when business trips brought him to my area. Eventually he achieved a long period of essentially pain-free recovery for over a year. But his symptoms did come back. Each time he sought me out in the office, by phone and later SKYPE, he seemed to improve. The reassurance from a physician who understood his pain was real, but his symptoms were benign. TMS was very helpful to him. He also went in and out of psychotherapy and patched up some issues at home.

I saw him recently on a visit to Los Angeles. He looked great, was very active and had lost weight with an exercise program. He insisted I do an examination of his back and a neurological examination. This activity almost ritualistically relaxed and reassured him. He could press on and be more physical in his life with less fear.

Lesson Seven: Mind-body pain keeps coming back until you are firm in your belief that there are no physical causes.

Jeff's case is important. One critique of some of the TMS books that have been published is that it seems most people get well very quickly, often miraculously so. My experience in treating between approximately 2,000 patients with TMS over the past twenty-five years is that some people experience that explosive recovery. Everything comes together for them and they improve rapidly and amazingly. I have also seen great, life-altering recoveries that take longer and involve more work on everyone's part, the patient, the doctor and the psychotherapist. People are different. Their minds, brains and emotions are unique. One size *does not* fit all.

This is the take-home lesson of this patient. If it takes longer, or more work, or has its ups and downs, TMS can still make a huge difference in your pain and in your life.

DEBBIE'S STORY

Debbie, a woman in her 40's, is a mom and a successful financial professional. She had been having a lot of stress with her company's money woes. She even considered a move to another state. She first experienced pain in her back. A doctor told her it was a "pulled rib" and she was prescribed physical therapy, which did help a bit.

Then she got scared by some things:

a) Her Achilles tendon became sore and her physical therapist alarmed her by telling her she was very sensitive to pressure in her legs.

b) Her internist frightened her further with a diagnosis of possible auto-immune disease.

c) She stopped her usual exercise program and began to worry more about the pain in her feet.

d) She returned again to the physical therapist who told her there was an imbalance in her body mechanics. A massage therapist told her she had trigger points.

e) She was not sleeping well.

f) She saw another specialist who diagnosed "tendinosis" of her ankles.

She eventually saw a foot specialist, a podiatrist, who told her that her x-rays were normal. Lab tests came back normal and disproved any auto-immune problems.

As I questioned Debbie, her Type T personality became more clear. She tried very hard to make everyone happy. She was a people pleaser. She told me she had had teeth grinding, bruxism and tension headaches at various points in her past. As for Debbie's childhood, her parents were great, but there were high expectations at home.

I examined Debbie and diagnosed her as having a clear case of TMS. The pain was a physical manifestation of her stress filtered through her personality style. She obtained a home-study program to continue at home. I saw her three weeks later. At this next appointment, she reported that she was much better and had taken it upon herself to read additional books on mind-body healing.

Debbie wrote me an email exactly two months after her first visit. This is what she said: "I am now completely pain free after following your program. I am a skeptic by nature and had I not gone through this process myself, I wouldn't have ever believed it possible."

SCOTT'S STORY

A while ago, a patient, who is also a friend, related his TMS struggle to me. I will call him Scott so that he can remain anonymous at his request. I mention that he is a friend because I was able to obtain some sequential information about his pain that is perhaps more detailed than I would have with a typical patient.

Scott told me that he was struggling with a personal health issue in his life and how it impacted him and his family. During this period, he began to have low back pain. Interestingly, back pain was not a classic TMS symptom for him. Previously, he had more tendonitis and irritable bowel intestinal related mind-body symptoms.

This time, he noticed low back pain and tried, as a well-trained TMS patient, to ignore it. This did not work, so he tried to talk himself out of it. This also did not succeed. Scott then decided to try some stretching to see if this would help. It did a little, but the pain kept coming back. To him, it seemed as if he needed more stretching.

Massage also helped, sometimes relieving the pain up to 90%. The pain kept coming back. He became more alarmed about his nightly pain, after reading that bone pain of the back, knee or leg which awakens you from sleep, can be a sign of a serious condition like a tumor or cancer. This did not happen every night, but it happened several times, and he brought it to my attention.

I planned to perform x-rays to reassure both of us that nothing was seriously wrong, but his schedule precluded that for a while. I discussed with him trying to "talk away" the pain when it occurred at night. This is a suggestion I often give my patients because it allows them to talk to the part of their mind that is creating the unnecessary pain. Surprisingly, for most patients, talking to their pain can often make it go away.

Scott told me a few days later that one night he woke up at 4 a.m. in a sweat with very tight back muscles. He recalled no specific dream, just anxiety. He told himself it was TMS and that the pain should just go away. He noticed it loosening up and quickly fell back asleep. That morning, he awakened without any pain or limitation of movement.

This is an example of how talking to your pain can actually make it go away.

But the pain did not go away for good. Unbeknownst to me, he decided to see a chiropractor near his workplace. The chiropractor had heard of TMS, fortunately, and did an examination that found very tight muscular trigger tender points, but no neurological findings or any bony tenderness.

The chiropractor reassured Scott that the problem was muscular and that one of two things would probably relieve it: 1) Deep tissue work, or 2) TMS treatment.

Scott later told me that hearing this helped him to relax a bit and the pain went away for a few days. But it did return.

Over the years, Scott had accumulated a lot of friends in health care and saw one of his physical therapist friends while he was traveling. This therapist friend did an examination and Scott was told of some weak muscles on one side, tired muscles on the other side and tight muscles on the weak side. Again, no sign of a bony, spinal or nerve problem was detected or mentioned. This reassured Scott even more. He left the physical therapist with a series of exercise recommendations, posture exercises and physical maneuvers that he could do to try to relieve the pain.

Over the next few days, he again had no pain. But it came back quite severely the day before he was to leave on a trip. This time, he decided to go back to the core mind-body message that he and I had talked about previously.

He told himself that three practitioners, me on the telephone, the chiropractor and the physical therapist, had all come to basically the same conclusion. There was nothing seriously wrong and he had tight muscles.

Scott began to understand the pattern of his pain. There was relief from the pain each time he was reassured of its benign nature. After some time had passed, there was a recurrence of pain. His tension and worry had built up again.

This time, he decided to "scream" at his mind/brain. He said to himself with strong intention, "Enough of this pain, I've had it. Go away!" This was an internal scream, but just as real as an external one.

This time it stuck. The pain went away within an hour of the scream and this time it stayed away. Scott went on his trip, dealt with his luggage and did not even need to stretch. He has now remained pain free for months. He is far more confident that he can keep the pain away indefinitely, or deal with it if the pain starts creeping back into his life.

Scott's story illustrates several teaching points, including:

Lesson Seven: Mind-body pain keeps coming back until you are firm in your belief that there are no physical causes.

That is why testing and physical examination has a role in the diagnosis and treatment of these conditions. Although the chiropractor and the physical therapist were not trained TMS practitioners, the careful exams they did helped reassure my friend Scott that he did not have a spinal tumor or disease, and that the problem was muscular or soft tissue.

This was crucial for him to be able to move to his TMS mindset of accepting the diagnosis and refusing to allow the pain to continue. This activated his helpful neural circuits, as I have described above, which stopped signaling the muscles and ligaments to contract and tighten via the brain and spinal cord.

Was his pain problem solved? It is hard to say for sure.

Sometimes this is all you need to do to move beyond the pain. Other times more emotional introspection is crucial to get at the core issue that is bubbling up and causing the pain problem. If introspection is needed, journaling, speaking with a loved one or close friend, meditation and speaking with a therapist, ideally one versed in TMS theory and treatment, are helpful. These steps help you get closer to the root cause of the pain and therefore you are more likely to find longer term relief.

JORY'S STORY

Jory and his mother came to the office one summer day. Jory was an athletic appearing young man who had played volleyball in high school. He was a college student, rising sophomore and not quite 20. Already, he had had two back operations. The first was a success and it gave him a few years of pain relief. The second did not help at all. He continued to suffer from a lot of leg pain. Several doctors, including the neurosurgeon who referred him to me, reviewed the imaging. He was not deemed a surgical candidate. There was no clear structural explanation for his persistent pain.

This neurosurgeon, whom I greatly respect, was open to the use of a mind-body approach with a patient such as this. His referral notes to me usually state, "Importance of mind-body relationships in chronic pain disorders... Experiential data and functional brain imaging..." This patient was open to other treatment options, curious, but hesitant, given his pain and disability. Jory was unable to exercise like he used to and felt like his body was failing him at a very young age.

His later high school and early college years included some disappointments, including relationship and school-related issues. He had a happy childhood, but was definitely a Type T personality. On physical exam, he had limited back flexion. He could only bend forward about 45 degrees. He had two of the six tender points that we look for.

I did diagnose him with TMS and advised he use the home study program. I saw him back about a month later. The pain had improved significantly with no medications or injections. Jory felt more than 50% better and when asked to bend forward, he nearly touched his toes. We talked a bit. I counseled him about aspects of his recovery and the study materials. He seemed more hopeful.

About a month later, our next contact was actually a personal letter to me, from his parents, on their family letterhead. The letter shared the joy of parents who felt they had "their son back." It described Jory as active with recreational sports at school, essentially living without pain and enjoying school a lot more as well.

I share this case with you for several reasons. First, it is incredibly gratifying and inspiring to be able to help a person heal, on multiple levels, and for them to literally get their life back. Second, this patient did really well without any psychotherapy and despite initial skepticism about the whole approach. Third, this patient had two prior surgeries. Fourth, he had recovered from chronic leg pain, which was present well over a year. So even post-surgical patients can, under the right circumstances have success. More on this later. No single case is typical. Every patient is unique. Here is a young person who did amazingly well. Other examples that are described will illustrate people who are in their late teens to their late 60's and above who use this method.

JENNIFER'S STORY

This patient has a wonderful, remarkable story. Jennifer was 25 when she first saw me. She played the cello at a very high level, but she had largely stopped playing music by the time she saw me in the office. She had a prior elbow surgery, cortisone injections and very little improvement after any of these treatments. Her symptoms had been there since her late teens.

When I saw her, any movement caused pain in her elbow, sometimes aching and sometimes sharp. Pain occasionally shot down her arm as well. She had to avoid driving because of the symptoms. Pain was worse in one arm but present at times in both. She did not know much about TMS, but was open to it from the little she had heard before seeing me.

Chapter VII, Instructive Patient Stories

When I saw Jennifer, she was working from home, doing clerical type work and teaching a little music as well. She had two of the Type T personality characteristics. She was a people pleaser and a perfectionist who pushed herself really hard. She had been playing her instrument since she was six and her life, for many years, had revolved around playing music.

She had tenderness in her lateral epicondyles, the soft tissue next to the elbow bone. She had three out of six TMS tender points as well. In the office, she was mildly tense. Jennifer did relate some childhood events of a sexual nature that were uncomfortable for her to discuss.

I diagnosed her with TMS and she left with the home program. I also referred her to one of the excellent therapists with whom I collaboratively work to help people with chronic pain. She studied the materials, thought about the office visit and what she had learned. She saw the therapist for four sessions of fifty minutes each. Remarkably, her pain was 50% better when I saw her a month to the day from her first visit and after two therapy sessions. She indicated that she was practicing talking to her pain, as we discussed. She was finding an ability to moderate or control it a bit.

Later, I learned that in another month her pain had gone away completely! She had a total of four or five therapy sessions. She can now play her instrument for two hours without pain.

What this tells us is that some patients, including those who have had unsuccessful surgery, who have pain in areas other than their back, neck or jaw, can have remarkable success if the correct diagnosis is made. They must be open to it and follow the treatment approach. In this case, seven years of pain was eliminated in two months. No surgery. No medication. No injections. This will not work for everyone, but when it does, what a benefit and what a joy for all concerned.

Take Home Exercise:

Do you see yourself in any of these examples? Why? What does this tell yourself about what you need to do next?

CHAPTER VIII

Do I Have TMS?

I designed the following questionnaire nearly fifteen years ago to give a guidepost to prospective patients and myself. I have included it in Chapter IV, but let us take a little time to dissect it. Our goal here is to help you understand what goes into the diagnosis of TMS.

The point scoring system and full questionnaire are in Chapter IV.

1. Have you noticed a relationship between your pain and your emotional state and stress level just prior to the onset of pain?

With this question, I am trying to ascertain if the patient, or prospective patient, has made an association between his emotional state and the onset of pain, a specific painful episode or the overall trend of pain. Specifically, I commonly find the major stressor may precede the pain. We can often find enough courage or adrenaline to get through a very challenging period. It often is right after that period of a loved one's death, the break-up of a relationship, a financial crisis or flunking finals, when the physical manifestation of that stress hits us.

2. Would you describe yourself in general as: Very hard on yourself, highly responsible for others, very thorough, orderly, a people-pleaser or a perfectionist?

Here I am trying to list enough of the TMS personality characteristics or traits to see if a person is aware of having these attributes.

Sometimes asking a spouse or loved one to help answer this question gives you a better answer than doing it yourself! Someone we are close to often sees aspects of our personality better than we do ourselves.

3. Have you suffered from other tension-related illnesses, such as:

- Hives, eczema, rashes brought on by tension?

- Spastic colon, irritable bowel, gastritis, reflux or heartburn?

- Tension or migraine headaches?

- Unexplained prostate trouble or pelvic pain?

- TMJ, teeth grinding or plantar warts?

Dr. Sarno first noticed this association and reported it in one of his early papers on TMS. Of these symptoms, the most powerful association I have noticed is irritable bowel syndrome. Tension headaches and TMJ are second. All of the others are about equal in connecting us to a TMS diagnosis.

4. Regarding the cause of your pain, have you been told that "There's nothing that can be done surgically," "There's nothing wrong," "It's a soft issue problem" or "The cause is degenerative changes?"

I try to get a feel for whether the patient has other diagnoses "floating" in their head or whether the patient is at a stage where the diagnosis of TMS, not yet made, not yet stated in other physician's offices, is a logical next step.

5. Do you spend a fair amount of time during the day thinking and worrying about your pain, researching an answer or obsessing about its cause?

TMS is not OCD, an obsessive compulsive disorder. It is very true that people with TMS, even more so than individuals with a variety of chronic disorders, do a ton of research on their condition. They spend a bunch of time every day worrying about what is wrong and what may have been missed. Not everyone is the same, but I have seen the most detailed, typed, organized medical histories and outlines of prior treatment from a lot of TMS patients. My office staff can see the TMS traits, just from the manner in which prospective patients ask their questions when making a first appointment.

6. Have you tried several different treatments or approaches for your pain and received only temporary or limited relief from each of them?

Very characteristic of the pattern of prior treatment is partial or temporary relief with many treatments and having tried many treatments before coming to be considered for TMS.

7. Do you find that massage helps your pain significantly or are you quite sensitive to massage in several parts of your back or neck?

This question attempts to find a preliminary way to tap into the TMS tender points before a medical exam. I felt that massage might be sensitive or provide temporary relief in TMS. I have included this question to capture something that otherwise must wait until a physical exam by a TMS practitioner.

Additional Questions:

8. Does the pain ever move to another location in your body or jump around?

This is the TMS migration phenomenon, also called the "Symptom Imperative" by Dr. Sarno in his earlier books on this subject.

9. Have you noticed the pain improve when you have another tension-related illness?

Again, this is symptom migration, substitution or distraction.

10. Has the pain significantly changed or gone away while on vacation, away from home or while distracted?

A vacation will not cure TMS, but for some people, the break from their routine allows them to relax, release some tension and be distracted from their worry. They feel a lot better.

Reviewing the above, you can begin to see some of the diagnostic factors that go into my making a diagnosis of TMS.

TMS DIAGNOSTIC FACTORS

What follows is another listing of TMS diagnosis factors, issues and findings that help me make this diagnosis in my office. Note that not all must be present. Some are more important than others.

Here we assume there is no structural or chemical issue to explain the pain.

a) Emotional stressors, factors and the timing of the onset of pain.

b) Personality Type: Type T characteristics.

c) Other prior psycho-physiological disorders are noted. In my experience, irritable bowel is the most powerful link, although a combination of tension headaches, TMJ and more, can also be a powerful connection.

d) Worrying about and researching causes of pain are very characteristic. Again, this relates to a Type T personality.

e) Childhood traumas, family discord and emotional wounds that have not healed are characteristic.

In my office, I listen closely to the entire narrative of the history of the pain problem. Careful listening leads to a better under-standing of the patient in the context of the pain. Clues may become evident as to emotional stressors, historical factors and personality types that contribute to the pain getting locked into a chronic pat-tern. Finally, the careful neurological and musculoskeletal exam tells me a lot. The presence of characteristic tender points helps confirm the diagnosis as well.

These tender points help confirm TMS but their absence does not rule it out as a possibility. These tender points overlap with a diagnosis of fibromyalgia, but are fewer in number and are not the most important part of diagnosis. (See illustration on the following page.)

Tender points are examined while the patient is lying face down.

a) One at each trapezius, the top of the muscle between the neck and shoulder.

b) One at the side of each lower back, coming from the side, the quadratus lumborum muscle.

c) One at each side of the upper outer gluteal region, the up-per buttocks muscle.

Additionally, there are two tender points, which can be help-ful. These are not of the original six as described by Sarno.

d) One at each iliotibial band, the upper part of the band, which stretches on the side of the leg from the hip to knee.

MAKING THIS DIAGNOSIS

Obviously and clearly, we cannot make a diagnosis in this book. I am sharing and teaching what I do in the office and the tools that I have created and assembled to get to the point of a firm diag-nosis.

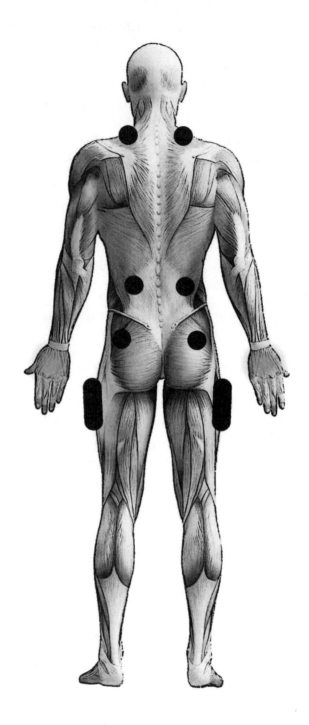

The TMS Tender Points

Let me review them again:

1) Emotional events, stressors, issues prior to the onset of pain (chronic pain)

2) TMS personality and Type T factors, tendency to "obsess" about the condition

3) Childhood issues, stressors, residual effects

4) A tendency to somatize emotions, to experience them in the body, prior to a problem, such as irritable bowel syndrome, headaches, TMJ and more.

5) Pain Diagram with multiple areas; this can be supportive, not required.

6) A surprisingly normal physical exam, OR a physical exam remarkable for extreme fear of movement or robotic-like movement, OR a physical exam that does not fit well with other findings, such as a normal x-ray.

7) The presence of two or more of the six major tender points. This is helpful, not required.

8) MRI or x-ray findings that are a) Normal, b) Normal variant, c) Typical wear and tear changes for age, d) Not consistent with location of symptoms or physical findings, such as the L/R switch.

9) Failure of multiple typical modalities and approaches. When one finds only temporary relief through acupuncture, chiropractic, physical therapy, epidural or surgery. Usually, three attempts are required.

10) The doctor's overall impression that this patient has psycho-physiological symptoms, after sitting and listening and observing and integrating the data.

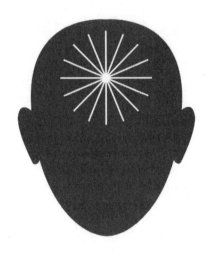

CHAPTER IX

Erasing Pain by Keeping a Journal

Why Writing about Our Pain Can Help

I realized many years ago that the process begins with a diagnosis in the office and needs to continue to be reinforced at home, to be even more effective. I advised patients to go home and keep a daily journal of feelings and emotions. Some did well with this advice. Others found it hard to sustain the effort of writing in a blank notebook after a few days or perhaps a week.

I wrote *The MindBody Workbook*, which is a guided journal that offers the reader daily questions, typically four, and a space for their answers. (1) Over the course of the 30 days of the workbook, people are asked questions that cover a variety of areas in their life, from their family, work, financial and childhood. These questions probe more deeply each week.

After the 30 day workbook is completed, I encourage people to keep writing, if not daily, at least two or three times per week. The style of writing is a free flowing, open association of events with feelings and emotional reactions to earlier experiences. If you are ready, you can begin this tonight, either in a blank notebook, on your computer or by downloading the *MindBody Workbook* from my website. Do not worry about punctuation, spelling or neatness. Look at it as a private journal that you may re-read, but that no one else is supposed to read without your permission.

I heard from a patient that some folks on the Internet were

referring to the *MindBody Workbook* as the "dreaded workbook." I think the dread that some people feel as they approach journaling about their life and their pain is the fear of opening up. For others, it is the discomfort of looking inside. Still others find the discipline of taking time out every day to write for 10 to 20 minutes to be difficult in their busy and chaotic lives. I am gratified that the workbook is not considered fluff and that it requires some effort. I find that just about everything worthwhile in life requires some effort.

Daily journaling can help reinforce a psychological thinking style and will help you to gain psychological insight. I find that learning to make this a regular part of one's thinking process occurs with daily or regular journaling about feelings and fears.

Take Home Practice:

Write about what happened in your life today.

Focus on anything that made you upset, excited, angry, joyous or frustrated. Let it flow out of you. Then write a little about your reaction to the event or person. Was your reaction similar to prior experiences with family or other relationships? How?

I return to the treatment of pain in the Twelve Stages of Healing in Chapter X.

This exercise is a good start for you.

Let me leave you again with Lesson Three, which is inherent in the Narrative Change that was described earlier in this chapter.

Lesson Three: Psychology and education can change the mind/brain and cure pain, not just manage it.

Chapter IX, Erasing Pain by Keeping a Journal

Some patients like to combine writing with drawing or sketching. This may help them to effectively express, define or describe their feelings. If you can sing about your feelings into a recording device or write a song, that can also be helpful.

For most of us, writing will be the clearest path to describing and defining your life situation and understanding your pain in a broader context.

A growing body of academic literature over the past twenty years or so has documented the benefits of journaling for particular conditions and for general health. As early as the late 1980's, Dr. Pennebaker started publishing on this subject (2) and believed that "Participants who wrote about their deepest thoughts and feelings reported significant benefits in both objectively assessed and self-reported physical health 4 months later, with less frequent visits to the health center and a trend towards fewer days out... owing to illness."

Australians Karen Baikie and Kay Wilhelm summarized the breadth of positive findings for "expressive writing" in an article they wrote. (3)

1) Fewer illness related visits to the doctor.

2) Blood pressure improvement.

3) Lung function improvement.

4) Immune system function.

5) Improved sporting performance.

There are lots of potential benefits. I have learned that my patients who journal, especially when they write about feelings and continue the effort daily, find it extremely helpful. For those who like the structure, the specific questions that I have chosen for the *Mind-Body Workbook* offers a more focused approach to learning about your psychological concerns and motives.

HOW DOES JOURNALING WORK WITH AND WITHOUT PSYCHOTHERAPY?

1) Some people will not or cannot see a therapist due to availability, cost or time. Journaling offers great emotional and pain benefits when you write about your feelings.

2) Some people do not believe they need to speak with a psychotherapist. After a few weeks of daily writing and journaling, they are surprised what comes up and decide to seek a referral from me.

3) For patients who are already seeing a therapist or just beginning, the daily writing is a great exercise to extend the therapy into the other six days of the week.

4) Journaling often helps the therapy to progress more easily because the patient has a wealth of material from their writing to discuss with the therapist.

5) When therapy ends, journaling remains a skill and a tool to continue to manage the emotional stresses and strains that inevitably come up in life.

WHAT DO I WRITE IN THE JOURNAL?

I encourage people to write about feelings and to write daily if possible. The ideal time is one when you can be alone in a room, without human or electronic distractions, for about 15 minutes. Start by writing about something that made you upset or happy that day. Yesterday if it is the early morning. Let the writing flow. Do not worry about grammar and punctuation. If your writing comes to a natural stop, reflect on your answers. Is there a connection here with your past? Your childhood? With writing you did in a prior week?

As you obtain insight, make an attempt to go beyond the expressive writing and make connections between emotions, pain triggers and the past. Finding patterns will add to your observation. If you are using the *MindBody Workbook* and find you have more to say about a particular question or subject, continue on another page or another blank notebook. If you are recording your thoughts on a smart phone or other device, that is fine too. It is important the feelings find a form of semi-permanence in written or recorded words rather than just thoughts. Research shows this to be more effective. (4)

HOW DO I DEAL WITH THE PAIN? I REALLY NEED TO UNDERSTAND THIS BETTER.

One of the most common questions I get is, "How do I really deal with pain? How do I do this "thing"?

Of course, I have different answers for different people, but let me share a few of these answers with you.

First of all, if you are having pain, it is important to ensure that the problem is not structural or chemical. If you have had a thorough medical workup and nothing serious was found, then you are safe to proceed.

Recall this:

Lesson Seven: Mind-body pain keeps coming back until you are firm in your belief that there are no physical causes.

The next step is to "talk to your brain." This internal dialogue is one of the ways that the brain rewires itself. Imaginary practice or mental imagery can rewire and improve the ability to perform tasks. An example of this would be practicing free throw shots in basketball. (5) Analogously, when you reassure your (emotional) brain that the pain is benign and offers nothing to worry about, you can make it disappear. Sometimes this happens right away. Sometimes it happens on the fifth try or the tenth. Sometimes there is a delay between the message and the response.

The key thing is the message, a calming, assertive, reassuring, "kick in the butt" conversation or phrase that tells the pain you are on to it and you are done with it. When people first hear about this, the process sounds like voodoo. When people first accomplish this, the result seems as if it were magic. When people become experts at this, they have learned a truly valuable skill.

Note that I describe the message with metaphors in the paragraph above that some might consider in conflict. What I am really emphasizing is that the individual style is going to vary from person to person in terms of what feels right and what works best. Some people need calming. Others need a jolt of energy. It is best to find your own style, using the general guidelines discussed. This is not one size fits all medicine.

Okay, so you have done the above. If you have succeeded, then the following is not relevant. If you have not, then do not consider it a failure. Consider it training for your future success. Most people cannot immediately stand up on the board when they take surfing lessons. Most people cannot pronounce a new language perfectly when they first study it. It is the same with this skill. It does take some practice, some adjustments in approach and some persistence to succeed.

But your pain is still there. You need something to do and something to take. My answer to this is that the mind-body method should be used first. However, we are all human and sometimes an ibuprofen or naproxen (Advil or Aleve) is helpful for the temporary relief of pain. Similarly, the solution to stress is withdrawal. Sometimes we need to lie down and take a nap, read or breathe slowly for a little while.

WHAT IS THE ROLE OF OTHER APPROACHES?

I am regularly asked about physical therapy, acupuncture and other approaches in the context of making a diagnosis of TMS. Let me address these therapies and the roles they can play, both negative and positive, in the treatment of TMS.

Patients typically come to me having tried, without significant relief, a long list of treatments. Often these have included acupuncture and physical therapy. Sometimes these modalities have provided temporary relief of pain.

What I typically tell my newly diagnosed TMS patients is:

• You have tried these approaches already.

• If they were going to succeed, you probably would not be here discussing TMS.

• TMS requires accepting a diagnosis and believing in this approach. (See Twelve Stages and Chapter X.)

• Therefore, it can be counterproductive to be doing too many things at one time for your pain.

• For time and financial reasons, I would re-focus your efforts on TMS right now. Take a break from the other approaches.

Usually, I can convince a patient to take a break from other approaches, at least for a couple of months, while we delve into TMS treatment and monitor response to it.

HOW ABOUT OTHER MIND-BODY METHODS OTHER THAN JOURNALING AND SELF-TALK?

I encourage my patients to find healthy ways to relax and cope with stress. Therefore, meditation, including mantra and mindfulness, is a reasonable option for many folks. Meditation can be as simple as sitting in a comfortable chair, in a quiet room, with the phones off and distractions blocked out. Close your eyes and notice your slow breathing. Think of a word such as "peace," "one," "truth" or something that is religiously or spiritually meaningful to you. Doing this for 10 minutes, gradually increasing to perhaps 15 to 20 minutes a day, can be therapeutic in many ways. Slowing down our nervous system in this hectic, frantic world is a benefit. Seeing one's thoughts drift in and letting them float away during the meditation may provide some distance and objectivity between your self and your thoughts.

Physical exercise is, of course, a great stress release. Walking, jogging, biking, swimming and other sports are all reasonable options. The key is to start slowly and to try to gradually advance your activity. You will become more confident in your diagnosis of TMS and the benign nature of your pain, where it has been advised.

Walking, in some ways, is the most meditative of all. Noticing the trees, gardens, clouds, squirrels, people and all the elements of nature and human life around you can be very soothing to your mind/brain.

Remember, TMS is not just stress control. It is insight and awareness. Of course, many people are already doing some of these things before they see a TMS doctor or read this book. The difference is the knowledge of what can cause your pain. Pain does not mean damage. The process of exploring emotional triggers, thoughts, feelings, stressors and personality factors in your journaling and your talking to a therapist, loved one or family brings great insight and awareness.

WILL MINDFULNESS FIX ME?

In my opinion, no. First of all, TMS therapy is a kind of mindfulness, although different than commonly discussed. TMS treatment teaches us to be aware of our emotional life AND its connection to pain and our health. Therefore we take something that we may have been ignoring and certainly not connecting, such as emotional causes, and link it to the pain. We do this explicitly in our writing exercises and in our minds for flare-ups and the relief of pain.

Simply doing mindfulness exercises, as are taught, is typically not enough. That is like being in psychotherapy with a non-TMS therapist. I have found that the combination of these very useful approaches, such as psychotherapy, mindfulness and meditation, AND the knowledge and connection that TMS thought and theory offers is the crucial combination to the successful relief of pain.

HOW ABOUT EMOTIONS AND STRESSES? ARE SOME MORE IMPORTANT THAN OTHERS?

Dr. John Sarno emphasizes anger in his books about TMS. I agree that anger, especially unconscious anger and anger from a disappointing or troubled childhood, are important emotions that can spill over into chronic pain. I tend to broaden this discussion to fear, grief and other emotions.

Some patients are more fear-driven. The pain relates to something they are afraid of or anxious about, for example, the fear of losing a relationship or a job. Another possibility is the anxiety of being successful enough or the ability to accomplish the goals they have set for themselves.

Grief, especially prolonged grief, is another important emotion. Grief is often about the loss of a loved one. Some people are more successful at going through the mourning and grieving process than others. Some emerge stronger. Others may avoid or be afraid of sinking too deeply into grief. This can lead to unresolved grief, which finds its way to the chronic pain.

Psychologists write about the "anger-in" and "anger-out" styles of the emotion. The terms are reasonably self-explanatory. The "anger-in" individual experiences internal arousal. The "anger-out" person slams doors and makes sarcastic remarks. As expected, being able to express anger "appears to lessen the negative impact of anger on emotional and physical function."(6)

The role of anger is accepted in psychology, in general, and specifically in the context of "pain" or headache. By the way, our goal is not to have people act-out their anger to be healthier, but rather to acknowledge it. Express anger through writing, gentle verbalization or release it with exercise.

For some patients, the issue is a disconnection from emotions. The term alexithymia is used in psychological literature to refer to individuals who have a difficult time identifying their own emotions. Consequently, they may be less successful at processing emotions than is typical. The word alexithymia is from the roots a = not, lex = word and thymia, which is feeling. These roots define a person who is unable to put a "word" or description to their feelings. We see patients, albeit a minority, who really struggle with this. Some of these folks are highly intellectual about their feelings and really disconnected from the affective or feeling part of themselves. Therapy can help this a lot.

An association between alexithymia and low back pain was reported in an article. (7) The authors looked at public transit operators, such as bus drivers or subway engineers, and found that those who had "difficulty identifying feeling" on the Toronto Alexithymia Scale (TAS-20) showed the strongest association between alexithymia and low back pain. (8) A total of 32% of these workers had low back pain during the prior 12 months. While treatment was not part of this study, the authors suggested that mind-body interventions "might have to appreciate these deficits in emotional awareness." Researchers looking at Chronic Fatigue Syndrome found a modest support for the alexithymia construct as a predictor of physical symptoms in this disorder. They also commented on "a defensive, high anxious coping style" identified in people with this condition. (9) This brief discussion reveals that patients can have different underlying emotional issues and makeup. The common pathways to healing, however, remain similar. Where appropriate, an excellent psychotherapist can help the patient delve deeper into these issues and tendencies. At its best, TMS therapy is practical, goal-oriented, plunges deep and re-surfaces quickly. It helps the patient avoid sitting too long in the emotional soup and baggage. The patient is motivated by the pain, learns fairly quickly from the interactive relationship and moves forward from his "stuckness" in the chronic pain state.

A patient wrote this a few years back:

"The Mindbody Workbook is a subtle masterpiece guiding one to oneself through one's anger. Such a journey in less delicate hands could be a frightening path leading more to anxiety than calm resolution. In following his gentle prodding guidance on this path of self-discovery through writing, I was led through anger, rage, judgment, rejection and emerged into calmness, forgiveness, surrender, acceptance and smiles. Yes, smiling just because that is how I feel at times. The weighty backpack of my past is much lighter now. New paths have opened to me to be walked and guided by a reuse of Dr. Schechter's workbook. May his guided journey lighten your load."

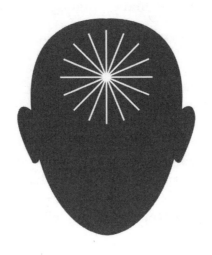

CHAPTER X

The TMS Twelve Stages of Healing©

For many of you, this will be the chapter that ties everything together and will guide you most directly on your healing path. This section and these stages are something I discuss with nearly every patient in my office that I diagnose as TMS. The process occurs toward the end of the visit, after the diagnosis has been made and helps the patient with pain to understand where they have come from and where they are going. This is a guide for how to get there.

1) Acknowledge that existing approaches are not working.

2) Become open to a new paradigm of diagnosis and treatment.

3) Evaluate the TMS diagnosis with an open mind.

4) Accept the diagnosis intellectually.

5) Accept the diagnosis in one's "gut" or heart.

6) Think psychologically, not physically or structurally.

7) Deal with your doubt about the diagnosis.

8) Increase your activity level.

9) Cope with flare-ups and the ups and downs of improvement.

10) Respond to friends and family about the diagnosis.

11) Deal with new symptoms from TMS in other areas.

12) Teach others to heal. Share your knowledge with others in pain.

STAGE ONE
ACKNOWLEDGE THAT EXISTING APPROACHES ARE NOT WORKING

As you are reading this book, it is almost certain that existing approaches to pain are not working for you. Perhaps they are working temporarily and you are seeking a more permanent solution.

By existing approaches, I mean medication, physical therapy, chiropractic, acupuncture, exercises and mindfulness. There certainly are a myriad of treatments available for back and other kinds of pain. I believe that the very existence of so many methodologies and epistemologies for back pain speaks to the lack of a single, successful and widely known treatment. After all, if everyone one were helped by medication, there would be no need for chiropractic. If chiropractic worked for all problems, why would some opt for massage? If exercise cured all back pain, then that would be all we need.

Getting some relief from mind-body pain using a traditional approach is not unusual. It is quite common. Many of these approaches are based upon returning the body to a normal state. For example, massage attempts to relax tissue and increase blood flow.

Chiropractic attempts to realign structural elements that are "out of alignment" and to seek a structural harmony for the spine. Acupuncture is derived from the Chinese medicine philosophy where "chi," or life energy, is believed to naturally flow through the channels throughout the body. A blockage in this flow leads to pain and ill health. Recent research suggests that acupuncture may affect how the brain experiences pain, but often only temporarily.

Medication focuses on inflammation or spasm. It attempts to relieve this at the tissue level and, theoretically, allow the body to then heal the problem.

I have utilized most of these approaches in patients with acute or new back pain or injury. Most of these approaches work, or seem to work, in people with acute or sub-acute pain. Another thing that works well is reassurance that there is nothing structurally wrong with the patient. A gradual return to usual activity is possible. In fact, this latter approach is often the most effective, clearly the simplest and most cost-effective. (1)

However, for many patients who are suffering from intense pain and have evidence of spasm, I advise medication, physiotherapy, massage trigger point injections or chiropractic. I also *emphasize* to the patient, "You are going to get better."

I RECALL BACK TO MY URGENT CARE DAYS...

I was one of several young doctors working the same, busy daytime shift at a medical clinic near the Los Angeles International Airport. It was not unusual for two of us to be reviewing x-rays, with a patient, at about the same time. We had one large view box that we tended to share, because it was the easiest way to show patients their x-rays. I overheard doctors telling thirty or forty year old patients, "You have arthritis in your neck," and "There are degenerative changes in your back."

While these terms are part of the medical lexicon, arthritis, or osteo-arthritis, is synonymous with wear and tear. Degenerative changes are wear and tear changes that are commonly seen in the aging spine and various joints in the body.

However, while technically correct in the most limited sense, I do not believe these physicians carefully considered the meaning of these terms to the patients with whom they spoke. A patient heard "arthritis" and often assumed the worst. "I'm not getting better."

"I've got arthritis, like my poor Great Aunt Jane." When a patient heard the more vague term "degenerative changes," he might have thought, "My spine is wearing away. How can I possibly get well?"

My review of x-rays with such patients were quite different. I would note, where appropriate, that they had some "wear and tear" changes. I typically would qualify this statement by pointing out that the wear and tear was "about what you'd expect for your age and level of physical activity over the years." I also would tell them the x-rays were taken primarily to make sure there was nothing significant in the bones like fractures or tumors.

The diagnosis of what is wrong with your back is a lumbar sprain, most common in an industrial setting, and "I expect you will improve and feel fine in a week or two." I believed then and I believe now that this initial reassurance is crucial to a patient's successful outcome from a back injury or neck pain.

Expectation becomes reality. Belief in what is wrong and how significant it is, or is not, is a vital part of that. The process of coming to accept an unconventional diagnosis is, in fact, a process. The vast majority of successful patients treated for TMS have not improved by first using structurally based, conventional or alternative approaches designed to "fix something that is wrong."

As a physician, I have come to accept this. Often, I have a strong feeling about people. From their first visit, I sense their diagnosis will be TMS. I certainly will ask about stress and tension and mention or emphasize its importance in their pain.

Sometimes my receptionist has a sense of who may be suffering from TMS. When she fields a call, the patient may have more detailed questions than a typical patient. The patient, a perfectionist, may come across as more worried about logistical details of the visit. Some bring a large, organized file folder to the visit! These behaviors reflect the outward manifestation of the Type T personality. (Chapter III)

However, it is rare that I get the kind of response that allows me to go immediately down that path. I plant a mind-body seed and hope that it will grow and germinate in the future. I also know that simple reassurance, a positive healing attitude and avoiding inactivity are enough of a diagnosis for most people to resolve their **acute** pain on their own. **Chronic** pain is, of course, another issue.

Each of the existing approaches is based upon a fundamental view that something must change in the person's structure or physical makeup. Physical therapy addresses a change in the muscles, posture or ligaments. Chiropractic seeks a return to a normal alignment or healthier state. Acupuncture speaks to a flow of "chi" akin to energy that is being blocked or impeded. Each of these philosophies implies that something external needs to be done to get well, by someone other than oneself.

Step One is to acknowledge that the approaches you have been trying so far have not worked to eliminate your pain.

STAGE TWO
BECOMING OPEN TO A NEW PARADIGM OF DIAGNOSIS AND TREATMENT

What does it mean to "become open?" A mind-body diagnosis represents a surprise, even a shock, to many people. They are familiar with structural explanations and they are quite surprised to learn that their emotions, brain or mind is playing a role, in fact the key role, in perpetuating the pain.

Openness is akin to readiness in the psychological model of how we change. It denotes a willingness to embark on a new path, to turn in a different direction, to hear something that could not previously have been understood.

Earlier in the book, I related my own story of the TMS diagnosis that Dr. Sarno gave me some thirty years ago. I was in fact surprised, perhaps shocked, when he said to me, "95% of this chronic pain is psychosomatic. What do you think of that?" But I was:

a) Desperate for relief of knee pain.

b) An intellectually curious medical student.

c) Familiar with the bio-psycho-social model from college reading.

d) Open enough to explore this connection.

A good number of my patients first were exposed to the TMS concepts by reading a book by John Sarno, others or myself. It was months or even years before they decided to apply the principles or seek a diagnosis. Why had they not done so immediately? I have heard the following:

a) "It didn't make sense at the time."

b) "The ideas made sense, but I decided to get an epidural instead."

c) "I wasn't ready."

d) "My wife was skeptical so I tried a different kind of acu-puncture."

These individuals were not yet open to a new diagnosis. They had the exposure, but not the readiness to confront their back pain problem in a new and different way. There is extensive literature on psychological change. Psychologists have written that there are stages of change: Pre-contemplation, Contemplation, all the way up to Readiness. I think there are analogous stages in recovering with TMS.

Individuals often have to get to a certain level of frustration or desperation. They need to be exposed to the idea of TMS at the right time, in order to explore the possibility that they are suffering from a condition that seems so different from what they had previously been told.

In addition, the diagnosis defines the appropriate treatment. If your problem is alignment, a massive disc or imbalance of chi, it makes sense to have appropriate treatments that affect these issues and correct them.

If your problem is TMS, however, then the logical treatment is to start thinking differently. At its core, the treatment is psychological, not structural. The cure is education, not more needles. Psychological insight is required, not more physical therapy or chiropractic.

That is not to deny that people sometimes improve with physical treatments, but for those who do not, becoming open means thinking "out of the box" and contemplating a larger view of health and disease.

STAGE THREE
EVALUATING THE TMS DIAGNOSIS WITH AN OPEN MIND

When an individual is open to a new diagnosis, she may be at a point when her mind is ready to look beyond the ordinary and to put aside preconceptions of what she has been told is wrong with her body.

For example, the media has perpetuated the "hard bed" mythology. For some years, it was believed that the firmer the bed, the more likely it would be conducive to good sleep and a healthier back. More recently, marketers have been selling the Duxiana bed and other premium brands, which no longer emphasize firmness as the only criterion for a good bed.

Similarly, an individual whose mind is open will evaluate the TMS diagnosis and determine if they see a truth and description for their pain. Does their pain get better with exercise or a massage? If so, this would suggest that something about physical activity, increased blood flow or perhaps the relaxing effects of these activities is therapeutic for them. Are they better on vacations or when distracted? Again, this speaks to a different solution than relief from a needle.

Certainly, respected physicians may have given a structural diagnosis to a person who suffers from TMS. The patient is inclined to accept this diagnosis until a point at which they are open to evaluating whether the diagnosis makes sense or whether it fits the facts. A different paradigm might make more sense.

It is important that the patient evaluating TMS have an open mind. They do not have to check their skepticism at the door, so to speak, but at least keep it in check so that it does not close one's mind to the truth.

STAGE FOUR
ACCEPTING THE DIAGNOSIS INTELLECTUALLY

When you confront this mind-body material, you are either attracted or repelled. In either event, you must decide if it is right for you. It may be intriguing, but not pertinent to your situation. It may be exciting, but not make sense.

The patients that go forward with this program eventually get to a point where they accept this diagnosis is valid and applies to them on a rational and intellectual basis. By this I mean that they understand that their pain could be caused by stress and repressed emotional issues. This intellectual understanding or acknowledgment in Step Four is in contrast to Step 5 where the acceptance is deeper.

Acceptance is crucial. For example, if you have diabetes, you can do a pretty good job of taking care of yourself by swallowing your pills, braving your shots and watching your glucose numbers. You do not actually HAVE to believe the diagnosis, if you choose not to.

With TMS, it is quite different. With a mind-body disorder,

accepting the diagnosis is crucial. With this acceptance comes change that is both psychological and physiological. Without it, doubt gets stronger and the tendency is to revert to the old way of coping with tension and pressure. The pain returns and the emotions are sub-merged.

In my office consultations, I explain that an intellectual accep-tance can be simplified to a list of pluses and minuses. The pluses are facts or evidence that confirm the diagnosis of TMS. The minuses are facts or evidence that do not support the diagnosis or at least leave substantial doubt.

To be more specific: An example:

Pluses:

a) I have the TMS personality.

b) My pain started right after a relationship breakup.

c) I am better on vacation.

d) My MRI shows nothing more than is typically seen in aver-age patients of my age without symptoms.

e) I have the typical TMS tender points when the doctor ex-amines me.

Minuses:

a) I always seem to have pain after getting out of a particular chair.

b) I am not able to play tennis the way I used to. It hurts too much.

In many cases, the minuses can also be explained within the TMS model, but again, we are trying to list every possible plus or minus so an objective, intellectual decision can be made. It is like buying a stock. They tell us to take the emotion out of it and make a decision based upon the numbers, the rate of earnings growth, the price to earnings ratio and stock buy backs. An intellectual decision is made.

STAGE FIVE
ACCEPTING THE DIAGNOSIS IN ONE'S GUT OR HEART

Reaching Step Five requires a deeper level of acceptance than intellectual understanding. This is the point when the excitement begins to fade and the connection to this diagnosis becomes calm and yet deep. At this stage, the doubts are slipping further away. They never go away completely. (See Step 9.) The belief in the diagnosis for TMS and its consequences are deeper.

Finally, when you viscerally accept and believe in this diagnosis, you can stop worrying and being afraid. You can channel your energy more constructively and not keep attacking yourself. You can learn more about your own emotional life and stop suppressing the portions of it that are dark, self-loathing and frightened. By acknowledging it all, you can be free of pain.

This is the level at which the fear abates and a calm may ensue. Much of the turmoil of the earlier stages has passed. The remaining work is then logical and doable.

How do we get to this level?

a) Read, re-read and immerse yourself in the materials available.

b) Reflect upon yourself, your personality and circumstances. Ponder the logic of this diagnosis.

c) A medical doctor, knowledgeable in TMS, can help greatly by looking you in the eye and giving you a clear diagnosis.

d) Look at your resistances, if any, and evaluate what is holding you back. Then get the information or support you need to bypass that block.

e) Take a leap of faith. It is safe and you can always go back.

STAGE SIX
THINKING PSYCHOLOGICALLY, NOT PHYSICALLY

This phrase, a variant on Dr. Sarno's original terminology, speaks to taking your focus away from the physical pain, the physical cause and the physical worry, and putting the focus and attention on something else: Your emotions.

When you focus on emotions, you also focus on your mind, your psychology and your feelings. This shift in focus, from physical to psychological or mental, is essential. For those TMS patients whose emotional lives are sufficiently complex, pain does not disappear simply by reading some material about TMS.

Thinking psychologically is not just about moving away from seeing more doctors, doing more therapy, visiting more practitioners and reading more articles on various mainstream treatments for chronic pain. Instead, it simply requires seeing how writing in a journal is part of opening up to yourself in an honest and caring way. It is acknowledging that your pain is at its essence a distraction from the emotional issues that are unresolved within you.

At this point, you can actually stop ignoring and repressing emotions and stop worrying. By the time you get a TMS diagnosis, you have done your due diligence and ruled out serious structural issues.

You now have discovered that the pain is not going to kill you and you have no structural malady or cancer. You are not sick. The pain is not structural or chemical. It is very real and it really hurts sometimes. The pain is just not happening for the original reason you thought. It is not a structural, medical issue. It is actually a psychological, TMS condition.

At this step, you can forget about the reminders that you have internalized to protect the body, such as never touching your toes or avoiding bending in a certain way without tightening one muscle or another. Relax and move fluidly. Let go.

It is time to fix the software. Another way of looking at this stage is to let the "hardware" feel and function properly again. Our mind is the software. Our thinking is the software. Our consciousness is the software. The hardware is the brain and the nervous system and the jaw, the neck, the back and the pelvis.

Nerve pathways are another way to look at the "Think Psychologically" imperative. Daniel Coyle's book *The Talent Code* and *Back in Control*, by Dr. David Hanscom are also helpful in this regard.

Pathways...

Following is a Diagram that I draw for patients. Here is how I explain it:

a) The person on the left is in pain and not happy. As their pain shifts into a chronic mode, the pathways, the lines, become thicker as the nerves and surrounding tissue speed up and solidify.

b) Note that the arrows go both ways. The brain and the body are feeding information back and forth. If you are in pain, it is the wrong kind of information. It is a vicious feedback loop.

c) Then you learn about this TMS approach. You are taught to focus on the psychological through journaling and therapy. You are encouraged to live your life, savor your relationships, enjoy your career and relax on a vacation.

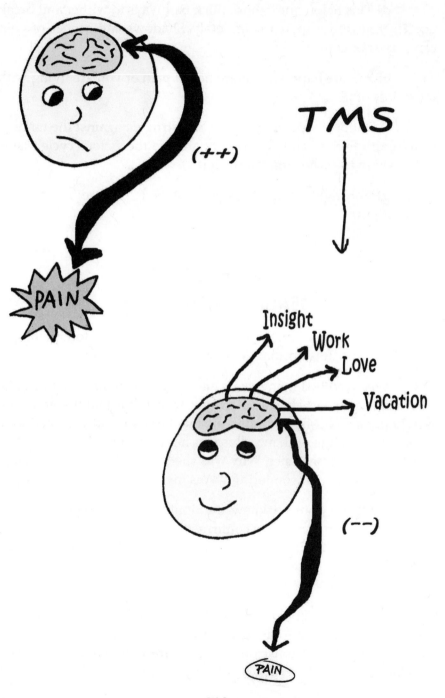

d) This helps cause those thick pathways to wither and break up. They never disappear completely. Shadows and echoes of pain can persist or come back.

e) You are happier. You are not in pain or you are living with much less of it.

f) Doubt creeps in. (Stage 7) You struggle against the tendency to return to the familiar habit of pain and the vicious cycle that is described in the schematic on the left.

g) You fight against this and succeed. You are a successful TMS patient.

STAGE SEVEN
DEALING WITH DOUBT

I have been writing and sharing lessons about doubt with patients for years. It is normal to doubt the TMS diagnosis.

I realized this many years ago when a patient called me. She had made a remarkable turn-around in her horrendous and long lasting pain. First, she reminded me that her pain had vanished for a week after meeting with me. This was her first pain-free week in two years. This astonished her. Why was she calling? The pain had crept back in and she was wondering, "Was my diagnosis really TMS?"

I felt her doubt. I knew the doubt was irrational. The two-week elimination of her pain confirmed my diagnosis. All it took was an office visit, a lecture and a workbook. I was 100% certain that her pain was benign and non-serious. Everything else fit to make the TMS diagnosis.

Why had the pain returned? Why was the patient experiencing doubt of the TMS diagnosis now? The doubt, I realized, was a mechanism of the unconscious mind to draw the TMS patient back into the prior mode.

The patient's prior adaptive style was to repress emotion and to create physical pain so that the patient would not pay attention to the emotional issues. Accepting the TMS diagnosis broke that pattern and relieved the pain. But if the patient was not fully ready to deal with her life and emotions more directly, then doubt could creep back in and try to turn her voyage around.

By being prepared for doubt and having a plan for dealing with it, you can prevent doubt from crippling your progress. The plan is: Accept the doubt. Acknowledge it. Understand that it is a trick of your mind. Instead of believing the doubt, you need to think intellectually and emotionally. Remind yourself that you have accepted the diagnosis and therefore, the doubt is meaningless.

Sit down and write a list of reasons why you accepted the diagnosis and why you believe in it. The doubt can fade away as you fight back against its regressive force. Move forward with a deeper acceptance of the diagnosis.

STAGE EIGHT
INCREASING YOUR ACTIVITY LEVEL

I am often asked, "So can I start running now?" A former runner asked me this because for three years he had not even been able to walk as much as two miles. But now that he was feeling better from his TMS work, he wanted to resume running again.

I told him, "Yes," but I urged a cautious approach for his return to activities. I held out to him the very real hope that he would be running soon. First, I wanted him to try fast walking and more journaling and more TMS-related reading and light jogging. When his acceptance of the diagnosis was stronger, he could try a short run and then gradually progress to longer ones.

Physical activity powerfully reinforces the model of TMS. It acts as a treatment amplifier in the sense of helping the patient to realize that the NORMAL we are talking about in our materials really means normal. It means a return to a full and active life.

So be more active! Start today, but get re-conditioned. Start slowly. Go faster as your belief in the diagnosis is stronger. If you get stuck, then take a leap of faith and go for a run after all.

Some of my patients heed my advice and cautiously proceed to be more active. One memorable case involved an athletic woman who told me she could not exercise for even ten minutes due to pain. I asked her if she could do five minutes. She laughed and said, "Yes, I can." I advised her to start with five minutes a day and add two minutes every third day. She came back three weeks later and was exercising 20 minutes without pain, more than twice what she thought was her "new" maximum. Her way of overcoming fear was to go slowly and get her confidence back.

Other patients have been given incremental advice in my office and chosen to go home and "go for it" on their own. Most choose this approach out of confidence in the diagnosis, the healing program and their own personality. Most do well. However, some flare-up with pain. This can be a setback that I try to help them overcome at a follow-up visit.

Whether you advance slowly or quickly, the point is to be less afraid and move. Do something and get your physical confidence back.

STAGE NINE
FLARE-UPS

Just as doubt is normal, flare-ups are natural as you are working within the TMS diagnosis. Pain relief is not a straight-line course. It is more jagged, like a lightning bolt in shape, with ups and downs. Accept this and understand that it is normal. A flare-up can mean several things, but it does not mean your life is ruined and the pain will be with you forever.

A flare-up can mean:

- A new emotional issue has crept in.

- There is continued repression of other emotional issues.

- Some sessions with a psychologist are in order.

The important thing for you to know is that having flare-ups, when the pain returns or shows up in another part of the body, is a normal part of healing from TMS.

Understanding that the flare-up will pass is part of the process of healing.

How should you respond to a flare-up, or for that matter, to TMS pain in general?

- Notice it. Then talk to it, attempting to think your pain away. "This pain is benign. It is TMS. It is from my mind/brain. I can control the pain and make it go away."

- Gently explain to yourself that this pain is not from damage. It is from stress and worry, from anger and fear. "I do not need it anymore. I am going to be fine."

- Some people benefit from screaming at the pain! "Go away TMS. I know what you're doing. It's my mind/brain that is the trickster. Enough with you. Farewell!"

Remember, this is new, so practice it and you will develop this powerful, portable skill of being able to think away your pain.

STAGE TEN

FRIENDS AND FAMILY

Now that you have changed your relationship with your pain,

your relationships with other people can change too. This means the people who have come to see you and relate to you as a "pain patient" may need to adjust to the new you. Just as you are adjusting to the lack of pain and your increased activity level, your friends, family and co-workers may need some time to adjust to the new you as well.

I mention this because you have been studying this subject and your friends and family likely have not. So give them a little time. Be patient. Perhaps even explain what you are going through so they can understand it.

Some relationships are based upon your identity as the "sufferer." You are the one who cannot do things because of your chronic pain. The new you may need a broader reconfiguration to thrive after you have gone through a TMS recovery, because you are not that person anymore. So be aware of this.

I encourage newly-diagnosed patients who are embarking on this healing program to change the subject directly, or indirectly, when people kindly ask them, "How's your back?" or "How's your pain?" For some, an indirect response like "I'm doing better, thanks" and a shift to another topic works well. Others prefer a more direct approach such as "Let's talk about something else. I believe it's better for me not to focus on my pain so much anymore. And I'm getting better anyway."

As you improve and are more physically active, resuming roles and tasks that you withdrew from is quite appropriate. "Wash the dishes!" I had this advice for one male patient with chronic arm pain (RSI) whom I was treating for TMS. He got some exercise with his arms that he had avoided for so long and I got big smiles from his wife at subsequent visits.

Lifting boxes and helping with luggage, might be tasks that you have avoided for a while. It may shake things up a bit, in a good way, when you resume these tasks. That is a good thing for you and your loved ones.

STAGE ELEVEN
TMS CAN MOVE OR CHANGE TO OTHER SYMPTOMS

TMS pain can move around. It is a tricky condition. For example, when patients tell me that their back pain is gone and they are mysteriously having a pain in their elbow, I deem that as progress.

Any change in the pattern of chronic pain is progress. It is your alertness to this movement or migration of symptoms that can help you cut them off and avoid a new TMS arena in your body.

The symptom migration often occurs just before the pain vanishes for good. The symptoms may not be the same kind of TMS you had before. For example, back pain can morph into jaw pain or headaches. Irritable bowel can switch to knee pain.

Stay alert to this. As with any new symptom that persists, have a doctor examine you. Be sure there is nothing structural or injurious. When you are sure, ignore the symptom or journal about it, or both. Get it to go away. You have the skills now.

Symptom migration is both a diagnostic factor in TMS and a factor in recovery. "I had irritable bowel in my 20's, tension headaches in my 30's and low back pain in my early 40's" is commonly heard in patient case histories.

The TMS migrates rather than disappears for multiple reasons.

a) Ongoing fear of a structural cause

b) Ongoing ignorance of the emotional issues in one's life

c) Doubting and not fully accepting the diagnosis of TMS

d) Needing more time to process the message of TMS and learn to master the method of healing

STAGE TWELVE
TEACHING OTHERS TO HEAL

There are many people in pain. Some have TMS, some do not. When you have recovered from TMS, do not become an evangelist telling everyone you know with pain that there is nothing really wrong with them and that all they have to do is learn about TMS and start paying attention to their feelings.

But do have a mission. That mission might be to share your story, your knowledge or your DVD or book with someone who could benefit. Many have been looking for help without finding something that works for them.

Do not push it because you will experience resistance, but be available. Be positive. Be open, but not overly prying. Remember, some people are not ready for the message. Some folks might enjoy a book on TMS as a gift but they may not read it for a year. Very often planting the seed is all you can do at this point. One must wait until the plant is ready to grow before watering it further.

For those of you who are helped or cured by this approach and have the skills in the following areas, your Stage Twelve could be more powerful.

• If you write a blog, you can mention TMS.

• If you work in marketing or public relations, you can help with making more people aware.

• If you work in healthcare, speak up for TMS. Bring a TMS speaker to your institution. It may be transformative.

• If you are affluent, there are non-profit opportunities available to help with research, build foundations and other efforts to study, educate and heal people with TMS.

• If you are a film or video maker, your medium is a powerful way to tell stories about success.

• If you are an Internet guru, the web reaches people all over the world.

Just offering a sympathetic ear to others and listening while gently guiding is often most appreciated.

THE THIRTEENTH STAGE?

What Do I Do Next?

Here I will discuss how to expand upon the Twelve Stages and utilize other proven techniques and approaches for pain relief.

AFFIRMATIONS AND SELF-TALK

Self-Talk and Affirmations:

A spiritual patient sent this to me some years ago. She had followed my instructions to write her own self-talk affirmations and this is what she came up with:

"Singing Joy Overcomes My Pain,

Divine Love overcomes my pain,

Holy breath within me overcomes my pain,

And all of these are gifts from the living G-d."

She concluded her letter: "Thanks for continuing to be a motivator for me. Another priceless gift."

Most "mantras" or affirmations are less spiritual, but I encourage people to write their own and this is what was meaningful to her.

Affirmations should generally be written in a positive and assertive voice. "I'm gaining control of my pain," or "I'm learning and growing stronger daily."

Affirmations for Anxiety

The words in parentheses are my additions. These affirmations are great for anxiety and many apply equally well to pain. (3)

1) Accept the feeling. It cannot hurt you.

2) Give yourself permission to feel anxious. (Pain)

3) Breathe slowly, through your nose.

4) Calm yourself with positive self-talk.

5) Let go. Float and flow.

6) Distract yourself. It is only anxiety. (Pain)

7) Use the adrenalin in a positive pursuit. Be active.

8) Do not let a bad day scare you. (A flare-up)

9) Give yourself credit for how far you have come.

10) Let time pass. It will go away!

In general, the best affirmation is one you create yourself. It should be affirmative, that is, positive in tone. For example, "My back won't hurt," is not as good as "My back feels strong."

PHYSICAL ACTIVITY, YOGA, ETC.

As detailed in the Twelve Stages above, physical activity is a part of the healing process from chronic pain and TMS. Patients often ask me, "Should I do yoga?" My answer is, "Do yoga, Pilates or other exercises that you enjoy to get your body moving!" Get back in shape. Many have lost conditioning due to pain, inactivity and fear of motion associated with the condition. **However**, I urge them to look at the yoga or Pilates as part of a fitness program and not as a treatment for their pain.

The reason is that we do not want the mind/brain to focus on the particular exercise or discipline as the cure. The understanding, the insight and your mind/brain are the curative agents. The exercise is to get moving, relax, increase blood flow and get stronger. If a TMS patient focuses on the exercise as the solution, they are likely to get a flare-up if they are unable to exercise because of their schedule, travel, flu or whatever life places in our way. The key is not to substitute a physical "treatment" for the core TMS model and program. Again, I do advocate exercise and a return to fitness for my patients.

PSYCHOTHERAPY AND PAIN RELIEF

What should prompt you to seek out a therapist to deal with emotional issues?

1) Journaling reveals lots of emotional issues you did not even realize were bothering you.

2) You had a particularly challenging childhood and some of these issues continue to affect your current actions and feelings.

3) You have been diagnosed with TMS or a qualified M.D. has excluded structural diagnoses AND you have read the books, done the home program and you are struggling to improve.

4) You have improved once before on your own, but it has come back and you need some extra help.

5) Your medical doctor feels that meeting with a therapist would be helpful for you.

6) Your significant other feels meeting with a therapist might

be helpful for you.

You do not have to be disturbed, crazy or flat on your back depressed to benefit from therapy for TMS.

What kind of therapy helps people with TMS pain? Ideally your TMS doctor would refer you to a highly qualified TMS therapist with whom the doctor has a great collaborative relationship. However, I understand this will not be possible in the majority of locations or situations for those who read this book.

Therefore, there are several options:

1) A relatively local TMS therapist can be found on a website, wiki or Google. Find someone who appears to have studied this subject and attended conferences.

2) A general therapist who is in your geographic area can help you with general issues that come up with journaling and self-talk. This individual is NOT a specialist in treating this condition or using this mind-body healing program.

3) A TMS therapist who works via phone or SKYPE from another city, state or country. This may offer those in certain geographic areas the best opportunity to have an expert work with them. The bang for your buck may be highest with a therapist familiar with TMS. Some are doing great work via the telephone, SKYPE and FaceTime.

TYPES OF PSYCHOTHERAPY

Years ago, Dr. Sarno described the ideal TMS therapist as "cognitive-analytic." By this he meant that TMS therapy involved both cognitive and analytic therapy. Cognitive Therapy focuses on changing how you think. You work on the elements of your thinking style that are counterproductive. Analytic Therapy offers a focus on understanding the dynamic issues in your personality and relating them to your childhood. This characterizes your emotional approach to stress and pain.

I have a broadened view of TMS therapy and therapists. I have worked with a lot of them over the past twenty years since I first met Don Dubin in Los Angeles. Don was the first TMS therapist for my patients. He was very devoted to helping people with TMS trying to heal. Like many great therapists, his approach was unique and included a goal-oriented focus on addressing the pain. He shared a lot of his own personal struggles and victories over TMS, and he offered a spiritual component as well.

Don's approach included an emphasis on "acceptance and surrender." By this, he meant to accept both the diagnosis and the individual who was as a TMS patient. Surrender to him meant that in order to "fight TMS," one had to first admit one could, temporarily, surrender to its power in order to understand it. Don's voice and ideas were recorded on the CD Number Three in The MindBody Audio Program. (2) Like me, his ideas continued to evolve after that recording.

Other therapists have incorporated Don's ideas and their particular training and background. TMS therapy, at some level, is good basic psychotherapy. Trust is important, a key factor in the ability to communicate to your therapist and vice versa. TMS therapy is different, in some ways, in that the TMS therapist should have the relief of pain as a goal that permeates treatment. This objective helps to make TMS therapy more goal-oriented than the sometimes open-ended nature of general psychotherapy.

Patients are often concerned about the length of time they may need for therapy. This will vary from person to person. Some people may find TMS relief in six to eight sessions, but continue therapy to work on other issues. Sometimes, in conjunction with, or following the home program and daily journaling, TMS therapy often achieves results remarkably quick. TMS treatment occasionally "flips a switch" in fortunate individuals, who are ready for change, primed for understanding and emotionally flexible.

For this reason, the growing use of Intensive Short Term Dynamic Psychotherapy (ISDP) has found its way into the TMS therapy community. Practitioners of this approach take a more gently challenging or corrective path. They share Don Dubin's active involvement in therapy, but focus on the patient's ability to obtain quicker results from a challenge to the emotional status quo. Supportive therapy plays a role as well, because going too fast at people's psychological defenses can be unnerving for some or lead others to seek another therapist. For the right person, ready for change, desperate for relief and willing to be open, this approach has shown dramatic results.

There are many schools of psychotherapy. Some behavioral components of therapy are being integrated into TMS therapy. Mindfulness meditation and stress reduction techniques have also contributed to healing in many individuals. A good therapist should not have an approach that is too formulaic. The good practitioner will have a bag of tools and apply the ones needed by the individual person they treat. However, some structure is beneficial. The goals of the therapy are relief of pain, accompanied by emotional understanding, insight and release.

CHAPTER XI

Research on TMS

MY RESEARCH

This chapter presents more evidence for the effectiveness of TMS as a diagnosis and treatment. However, research is not interesting to everyone. You, the reader, are not in school, so if you wish to skip this chapter, that's fine. You can always come back to it later.

In addition to providing proof of the treatment approach, TMS research also reveals much about the challenges of the field. In fact, I was feeling frustrated at the lack of interest and acceptance for TMS among the medical community in the early 2000's. With the help of a generous patient's family foundation, the Seligman Medical Institute was established in 2003. For approximately four years, I had access to funding that allowed me to hire a colleague, Arthur Smith, Ph.D., part-time, as well as research assistants and consultants when needed. Despite this opportunity, as you shall see, we were still limited in our ability to achieve our more lofty research goals. Research costs a lot of money and takes a lot of time to do well.

STUDY OF RESPONSES TO TMS MATERIALS

We started modestly with a postcard style questionnaire that looked at results from the home educational materials ordered by 200 individuals from the website, www.MindBodyMedicine.com. The study was very limited in that it was not *randomized* or *controlled* and the response rate to our mailing was approximately 18%. While this is a well above average response rate for this type of mailing, it is too small a response rate to draw definitive conclusions.

Of the 37 respondents, 28 (76%) felt that the materials were "a lot" or "tremendously" helpful. Seven (19 %) felt the materials helped "a little." Only two (5%) felt the materials were not helpful at all. 23 (62%) respondents felt that the materials had helped them heal "a lot" while three (8%) felt the materials played no part in their healing process.

Of the five individuals (13.5%) that had seen a TMS-oriented physician, four (80%) indicated that their problem was "gone" and three (60%) felt the materials helped "a lot" in their healing process.

This "Web Orders" research was not deemed publishable by the first couple of journals we submitted it to. Partially this was due to the lack of awareness of TMS and its treatment. Mostly this was due to the lack of scientific rigor of this form of research. Looking at the people who did respond, it is clear that the TMS program, even a home educational program obtained from a website, can have a highly significant effect on a sub-population of pain sufferers.

This article, while never published as a whole, was cited in another article I was asked to write for *Practical Pain Management*, entitled "At Home Educational Materials For Chronic Pain." (1)

FIRST OUTCOME STUDY

Our research team next compiled data from a study partially completed before the foundation's funding began and wrote a paper on this re-analyzed data. Again, we ran into obstacles based on the study design and outcome measures utilized, as discussed below. The research was eventually presented as an abstract at the American Psychosomatic Society (APS) in 2005 and was published, as an abstract, in *Psychosomatic Medicine* online. (2) I traveled to Vancouver with Dr. Art Smith in order to attend the conference and present our abstract.

This study utilized a trained research assistant who attempted to contact 107 former patients treated for TMS. Utilizing a telephone questionnaire, their current levels of pain, medication usage and related factors were analyzed.

FIRST OUTCOME STUDY RESULTS

Shown in Figure 1, the overall results were as follows:

44% (38 patients) were classified in Outcome Group A. These patients were living essentially pain free and taking no pain medications, other than occasional over the counter (OTC) remedies.

17% (14 patients) were classified in Group B. These patients had some pain, pain that does not rule their lives, and took little or no medication.

18% (15 patients) were classified in Group C . These patients had shown some improvement, but were still having pain and some restrictions. They took some medication.

21% (18 patients) were classified in Group F. These patients, who had no effect of treatment, were still having pain, impairment and still using medication.

This study appeared to show that 61% of the treated subjects had excellent or very good results (A and B) and about 21% were not successful at all. While highly significant clinically in a chronic pain population, this data had many limitations from a scientific standpoint. Also, I felt that my treatment method and materials had developed further and that my results would be more impressive if we studied a more recent group of patients.

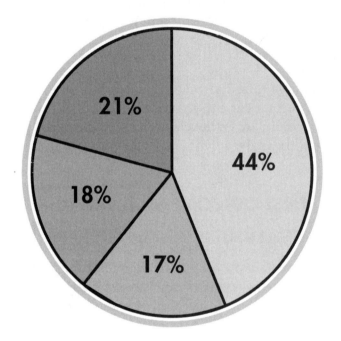

Figure 1

We learned that this classification system, while logical to us, was not as clear to journal reviewers who preferred standardized outcome measures such as Visual Analogue Scores (VAS) and Quality of Life Measures (e.g. SF-12). In order to use these measures to compare outcomes from beginning to end of treatment, advanced planning in our clinical intake process was required to ensure additional forms were completed prior to or at the first office visit.

DISTRACTION PAIN SYNDROME PAPER

While developing our next research study, we had an opportunity to write and publish a theory paper describing the mechanisms for TMS, or what we called Distraction Pain Syndrome (DPS). This was published in *Evidence Based Integrative Medicine* in 2005. (3) While the nomenclature has not caught on, my patients find the terms DPS easily understandable and useful as they analyze their own painful condition.

SECOND OUTCOME STUDY

We continued to refine our research design, affiliated the Foundation with a University based biostatistician, Stanley Azen, Ph.D., (University of Southern California) and did another telephone and email based follow-up study, again non-randomized and non-controlled, which was a case series study of patients treated in my office during a two year period. This study used the more formalized and accepted outcome measures like the Visualized Analogue Scale (VAS) and SF-12 scores, statistical measurements of psychological and physical overall health.

This study was published in the prestigious alternative or integrative medicine journal, *Alternative Therapies in Health and Medicine*, in 2007. (4)

SECOND OUTCOME STUDY RESULTS

Our results were excellent, in spite of the long average duration of pain from which the chronic pain patients suffered prior to diagnosis.

"The majority of participants were male (63%); the average age, 46 years; and the average duration of back pain, 9 years." (4)

After TMS mind-body treatment, mean VAS scores for "average" pain decreased from 64 to 30 (p<0.0001). Mean scores for "worst" pain decreased from 89 to 58 (p<0.0001), and for "least" pain, from 35 to 12 (p<0.0001), representing VAS score reductions of 52%, 35% and 65% respectively. In addition, there was significant improvement (average increase = 9 units) in the Physical Health composite score of the SF-12 (p=0.005). The Visual Analogue Scale is a 100-point scale, divide by ten for the "ten point scale equivalent."

"Medication usage decreased significantly with treatment (p=0.0008). Notably, of the 19 participants who regularly took medications pre-treatment, 13 (68%) never or occasionally took medications post-treatment."

Activity level increased significantly with treatment (p=0.03).

The data clearly showed that the program helped people with chronic pain achieve statistically highly significant reductions in pain. As noted above, the average duration of pain in the participants was nine years. The results were comparable to or better than other studies that involved long-term treatments and highly expensive or intensive interventions. Medication usage decreased, while activity increased.

Because we did not have a *control group* to compare our results to, we decided to compare our outcomes to published studies of response to other treatments for chronic pain. This data would be helpful. Some of these other efforts involved far more intervention, more expense and more treatment and still had less benefit to patients. (4)

More details are available in the original published papers and are referenced on the Seligman Medical Institute website. See the publications section at www.smi-mindbodyresearch.org.

I have taken a break from active research on TMS at this time, while focusing on clinical practice, writing and study. The future of TMS research clearly needs randomized controlled trials and university-affiliated research. Sources of funding may include the National Institutes of Health alternative medicine division. Private funding from a larger foundation may also prove to be a source of backing for this kind of research.

CHALLENGES OF HIGH-QUALITY MIND-BODY RESEARCH

Again, the challenges of mind-body research are multiple:

1) A TMS study requires more complex interventions than a pharmaceutical study that involves comparing groups of participants taking an "active pill" versus an "inert pill."

2) More intricate study designs are required or needed to prove the hypothesis.

3) In general, an infrastructure is needed to do the research.

4) There is the expense of finding, recruiting and randomizing patients and then diagnosing, treating and following them for a suitable interval.

I anticipate that other TMS doctors and those with interest in alternative approaches to chronic pain will pursue additional research. If the combination of funding and time presents itself again, I would enjoy being part of additional research on TMS, including functional MRI imaging to see the brain and its changes during TMS treatment.

OTHER DOCTOR'S WORK

John E. Sarno's Publications in This Field

Dr. John Sarno began writing about pain and the mind/emotions in the late 1970's. His early papers include "Psychosomatic Backache," published in 1977. (5) In 1981, he presented "Etiology of Neck and Back Pain, an Autonomic Myoneuralgia." (6)

He most recently published a paper with Ira Rashbaum, M.D., in 2003, entitled "Psychosomatic Concepts in Chronic Pain." (7)

Dr. Sarno's papers included presentations of theory, clinical descriptions and also a psychodynamic paper with Stanley Coen, M.D., titled "Psychosomatic Avoidance of Conflict in Back Pain." (8)

He is most well-known for his four books on pain. (9, 10, 11, 12) I was fortunate to be acknowledged in his first book for helping to edit the work and for my efforts to perform a follow-up study, under his auspices, that is cited in that first book and subsequently in his seminars for many years. At least two of these four books were best sellers and are sold internationally in many languages.

Howard Schubiner's Publications

Dr. Howard Schubiner has been active since becoming aware of the TMS diagnosis and treatment approach. He published, "Pain and Emotion: a Biopsychosocial Review of Recent Research." (13)

Schubiner has been working under a larger fibromyalgia grant and with his colleagues had published a randomized clinical trial (RCT) entitled, "Sustained Pain Reduction Through Affective Self-Awareness in Fibromyalgia: A Randomized Controlled Trial." (14)

The study consisted of 45 women with fibromyalgia who were randomized to treatment or who had not yet received treatment. The intervention began with a one-time physician consultation, followed by three weekly, two hour group sessions based upon a mind-body model of pain. Sessions were focused on structured written emotional disclosure and emotional awareness exercises.

Results, as reported: The intervention group had significantly lower pain severity (p < 0.001), higher self-reported physical function (p < 0.001) and higher tender-point threshold (p = 0.02) at six months compared to the control group. From baseline to six months, 45.8% of the ASA intervention group had ≥ 30% reduction in pain severity, compared to none of the controls (p < 0.001).

The research group concluded: This study suggests the value of interventions targeting emotional processes in fibromyalgia, although further studies should evaluate the efficacy of this intervention relative to active controls.

Dr. Schubiner also published a case report entitled, "Recovery from Chronic Musculoskeletal Pain with Psychodynamic Consultation and Brief Intervention: A Report of Three Illustrative Cases." The report described, "Three cases in which various types of chronic musculoskeletal pain were successfully treated using a small-group psychological workshop combined with a single consultative session." (15)

FUTURE EFFORTS

Clearly, there is a need for larger scale studies for patients with back pain, arm pain, fibromyalgia, TMJ, headaches and other disorders. At least a step or two in this direction has begun. An appropriate criticism of TMS theory has been that the treatment and theory expanded without scientific studies to back it up. While this may be true, Dr. Sarno's focus during his long career, my own and those of my colleagues in this area, have been primarily treating patients.

Clinical research tailored to the highest standards of modern science takes a lot of time, money and personnel. We are not academicians with large research teams behind us. Typical funders of research such as pharmaceutical companies are not interested in this kind of non-pharmacological treatment.

This does not excuse the lack of double blinded, randomized controlled studies but it does explain the focus of our TMS community on treatment. Research is something several of us have done, but more time and resources are needed to provide more scientific evidence for this powerful and important work. As for practical evidence, see Chapter XII, Patient Stories That Inspire.

CHAPTER XII

Guidance for Physicians and Healers

Very few doctors and healthcare professionals treat chronic pain. Practitioners in the field of Orthopedics, Family Medicine, Physical Medicine, Neurology, Sports Medicine, Rheumatology, Chiropractic, Osteopathy, Acupuncture, Physical Therapy and Massage Therapy treat millions of patients every year, but only a few seek a diagnosis for chronic pain.

A large number of practitioners are treating conditions that can be defined as psycho-physiological. Up to 90% of depressed patients may present physical symptoms and conversely many physical symptoms are due to psychological causes. (1) Healthcare professionals must realize how many patients are dealing with stress and how much it is affecting their health and bodies.

I have included this section for physicians and health practitioners to begin teaching them an approach that can help with their chronic pain and psycho-physiological disorder patients. Many of them find these individuals particularly challenging to care for. With the methods taught in this book, their practice can be more satisfying and their outcomes will improve.

What follows is a letter I have previously written to physicians who inquired about this method of healing.

TMS: A LETTER EXPLAINING THE DIAGNOSIS AND TREATMENT

Dear Doctor,

Among the many diagnoses and treatment approaches that I use in my office, the primary one for chronic pain is Tension Myositis Syndrome (TMS). This diagnosis was developed over 35 years ago by John Sarno, M.D., Professor of Rehabilitation Medicine at NYU's Rusk Institute.

The diagnosis is not widely known in the medical community. There are several reasons for this, including a lack of published data. Also, medicine has a pronounced reductionistic focus that has historically developed and been quite successful, especially for acute disease processes.

At its essence, the diagnosis of TMS is a description of the cause of back pain, neck pain, tension headaches and TMJ. This logically leads to a specific treatment approach. The diagnosis implies that the physical pain experienced by the patient is in fact a manifestation of psychological tension and is therefore most effectively treated with a psychological focus. In more contemporary neurobiological terms, the pain is centrally based and enhanced by amplifying descending pathways. The treatment is to focus on the individual's perception of pain to modify the inhibitory descending pathways to reduce and eliminate pain.

The pain may manifest physically as a muscular spasm, soft tissue pain or even involve a minor neural component, such as tingling, when it is NOT primarily due to a structural process in the spine or other structures. For this reason, it is essential to exclude structural lesions, such as large disc herniations, nerve compression, severe stenosis and tumors, before making this diagnosis. I recommend a careful neurological examination.

The diagnosis is typically made in patients for whom multiple attempts at physically based treatment have failed. I refer here to physical therapy, chiropractic, acupuncture and even epidurals. There are two reasons for this. First, patients rarely consider a psychologically-oriented diagnosis for physical symptoms until they have first tried conventional and alternative approaches to treating that pain physically. Second, patients typically find their way toward a TMS-oriented doctor when they are desperate, often after the failure of multiple approaches.

Diagnostic criteria for this condition include:

1) Excluding structural pathology. (NB: minor disc bulges do not rule out TMS as the actual cause of pain.) MRI's are often over-read and must be interpreted with care to ensure an accurate diagnosis is made.

2) Characteristic personality issues, such as perfectionism, being hard on oneself, being highly responsible, often meticulous and thorough.

3) Other psychosomatic conditions in history, such as IBS, tension headaches and stress-induced rashes.

4) Pattern of psychological crises before or during attacks. Anger, grief and fear.

5) Tendency to over-restrict activity based upon pain or based upon faulty advice from prior practitioners. 6) Characteristic tender points.

Treatment includes:

1) Making the diagnosis and having the patient buy in, accept, and believe in the diagnosis.

2) Teaching the patient to "think psychologically" about the pain, not to focus physically and therefore not fear physical activity.

3) Educational materials and *The MindBody Workbook* for home study use are available.

4) Cognitive-based psychotherapy where indicated. More severe, long-standing cases and people with troubled childhoods, such as molestation, are often referred.

5) Follow-up visits with a practitioner to assess response and fine-tune the program.

6) Gradual increase in activity level to normal is important.

We find that the belief in the diagnosis is crucial to success with this model. The patient is undergoing a change in their belief system about the pain that causes dramatic physiological changes leading to an interruption of the pain-fear-spasm cycle. This does not occur until the patient accepts the diagnosis, reduces their fear and worry and begins to re-focus psychologically. The shift in attention is consistent with a reversal of the chronification process that appears to occur in the brain when acute pain from trauma or injury, becomes emotionally linked and chronic. Functional MRI imaging studies have demonstrated some of these changes. References are available.

The success rate in patients, who are diagnosed with TMS and follow through with treatment, is quite high. Follow-up studies have demonstrated 60-70% success (or higher) without medications or physically based treatments. The cost to the patient is quite reasonable. The program is non-invasive and safe.

Note that this program is not the behavioral management of pain. The diagnosis and treatment is predicated upon the likelihood of the elimination of pain by the interruption of the psycho-physiological pathways that have become the pain problem itself, whether initially the cause or merely the perpetuating factor.

Yours truly,

David Schechter, M.D.

WHAT WILL IT TAKE FOR A PHYSICIAN TO RESPOND TO SUCH A LETTER OR TRY TO UTILIZE THIS APPROACH?

• Openness to a different viewpoint. A broader perspective on health and healing.

• A feeling that current methods are incomplete or not fully successful in many people.

• Personal experience or contact with a close family member, a friend or a patient who has been helped by the TMS method, is helpful.

• A bit of courage and energy to explore the unknown. To become familiar with a process that one was not initially trained in.

What mechanisms can a healer follow to learn more and develop skills in this area?

• Read this and other books on the subject of TMS.

• Find doctors doing this work and seek a mentor. (See www. MindBodyMedicine.com/doctors.html and other listings throughout the Internet.)

• Take the first step with a patient. Find a suitable patient and suggest they read one of the books on this subject. A person open to this treatment will be more easily guided and healed with a mind-body program.

• Do not be discouraged if there are challenges or an initial lack of results.

I am open to speaking to physicians and other healers one-on-one by phone or online video calls. I am also willing, if there is sufficient interest, to developing physician training. A visit to my office and seeing a couple of patients with this disorder and watching how I treat them is another option. I may develop more video of actual patient encounters, with appropriate consent, for teaching purposes.

I believe that there are other TMS physicians who might allow you to join them, if requested. We can help coordinate that as well.

CHAPTER XIII

Inspiration from Thankful Patients

I hope these comments will be helpful to people with pain that are seeking inspiration from those who have succeeded in relieving their pain, and to health care practitioners who are looking to become healers of pain, as well.

Re-reading these testimonials gives me goose bumps and reminds me that the day-to-day struggles are worth the effort, because lives are changed with this approach.

The correct diagnosis leads to the correct treatment. There are so many people who do not receive the TMS diagnosis for their benign chronic pain.

• • • •

"I am writing to express my thanks for helping me achieve what I had previously given up hope on. As you know, before I saw you I had severe back pain and had experienced frustrating episodes of plantar fasciitis and patellar tendinitis dating back to high school. Now I am completely pain free, and I know that I have been cured for good.

"Now, instead of spending my time doing worthless stretching and back-strengthening exercises, I jog or play basketball at least five days a week. I no longer worry about my posture (I'm slouching in my chair as I type this!) I disposed of my orthotics, which will save me about $200 every other year. I also got rid of my various back pain devices (magnets, gravity boots, braces, etc.) Now, I rarely even think about my back or my feet, except when I remember that they once dominated my life. Occasionally, I will get a brief episode of pain, but I am able to ignore it and it usually goes away within a day or two, if not a few hours. It's amazing how quickly pain can leave your body when you no longer fear it… Dr. Schechter, I owe you a tremendous debt of gratitude."

~ J.H.

"I also just wanted to thank Dr. Schechter again because it is thanks to him giving me the correct diagnosis of TMS that I have been able to work full time again for the first time in 12 years! What a joy… Thank you for your important work, it changes people's lives!"

~ Lisa E.

"Horrible, debilitating pain, no concrete diagnosis, all tests normal, unable to work, walk or sit, tried everything from ortho-pedists, physical therapists, hip specialists, surgeons, chiropractors, healers, body workers, juice fasting, detox, meditation, prayer, vi-sualization, positive thinking, etc. All really to no avail. The book, workbook and DVDs are my lifesavers!"

~ A. C.

"I am writing to you, because I think you are a real hero and I want to help you help others in whatever way I can. I believe my own story is amazing and can help others.

"I drove up to see you from San Diego for a TMS consult… My consult with you was excellent and took me to the next level in the Mind-body healing paradigm."

~ K. I.

Chapter XIII, Inspiration from Thankful Patients

"I was a patient of yours back in 2001 and visited you in your then Beverly Hills location. I had been diagnosed with a herniated disc and after every treatment from chiropractic, orthopedic, cortisone shots and finally had been told that surgery was the only hope. My lower back pain was chronic and debilitating. I was one of those who heard about TMS via Howard Stern! Anyway after visiting you and completing your program I became pain-free and that has been the case for the past nine years. In that time I have been active (even doing Taekwondo!)"

~ J.G.

"With Dr. Schechter's clearance, I returned to work in October 2003 and I'm at work since then. I still have some symptoms or limitations, but I can function well with housework at home and software engineering job at work. Compared to the total disability status before seeing Dr. Schechter, I am glad for the results and am really thankful that I found Dr. Schechter to treat my condition.

"Based on my experience I believe that RSI is TMS or primarily due to TMS. If one has RSI symptoms that don't get any better after a couple of months of rest and treatment, he should give TMS method a serious try. If he grasps the TMS concept and gets better immediately, that's great. (If you search the web, a lot of people completely recover very soon after trying TMS.) But if you need some medical support and help like me, there are TMS doctors like Dr. Schechter are there to help. Keep trying the TMS approach and you'll get better, that's my experience."

~ J.E.H.

"I just wanted to thank you for you tapes and workbook- they are excellent! I read Healing Back Pain, and lost 90% of my pain, but still had occasional flare-ups, and some fear. The workbook really helped me stop the flare-ups, pin point a couple of things at work and while driving (road rage) that caused the flare-ups. Thanks again."

~ A.J.

"The pain is completely gone! There are times when I notice it here or there but I just acknowledge whatever is going on and in minutes I'm fine. I just wanted to thank you for giving me my life back. I thought I would never be free from back pain. I've done all I can to spread the word about TMS and the books. I feel like if it could help someone like it has helped me then nobody would have back pain. After two years of almost no activity I am back to walking, riding my bike, doing aerobics, etc. I am a complete believer in this thing called TMS."

~ K.P.

"My TMS is still here but I've managed to control it with moments of flare ups here and there. Over the past year, I've faced some difficulties with schooling and some relationship problems, which I know are the causes of my pain but I've managed to control and fight it. Just thought you wanted to hear this story. If there is anything I can do to help, please don't hesitate to ask. I'm always willing to help you as well as any other people you think I can reach out to. If there are any patients, please refer them to me and I would be happy to talk with them. Take care."

~ E.L.

"I just wanted to write and let you know how fantastic I am doing. My pain is almost completely gone. I just get a little sore and achy after exercise, but I am confident I am on my way to getting my TMS under control and living a normal life again. I had my last appointment with Don today. After my last follow up visit with you, my psychotherapy session with Don Dubin (Authors Note: retired) was priceless. I uncovered some deeply buried emotional feelings I never knew I had and shortly thereafter, the pain started leaving my wrists and my ankles. I am free of pain.... Thanks for all your invaluable guidance and help. It is still so hard to believe that after 5 years of chronic pain, that after 6 months of putting the TMS theories into practice, I am free of chronic pain. If there is ever anything I can do to help others suffering TMS, please let me know."

~ K.D.

"Before he saw you, he was in pretty bad shape. It's so wonderful how you were able to treat/help him. I'm always here to help you because I really believe you do wonderful work."

~ K.B.

"Over the past few days I have watched your DVD and listened to your CDs and I have been CRYING AND WALKING at the same time. IT HAS WORKED!!!

"I made an immediate connection to emotional events in my life, to each of these painful symptoms. Over the years, I have had back spasms, left wrist pain (I had to wear a wrist guard), left foot pain and now my left knee. After reading about TMS a few days ago, I can still feel pain in my knee, BUT I have lost my fear. My pain has been reduced and I feel so excited. Can this be true????????? Can this really work for me??? I feel so uneasy at how fast it has worked. Is it possible? I am scared!!!

"I think my knee is linked to not being able to work in Hong Kong. (Insecure, Guilt, Anger etc.) Now that I know about TMS, I feel free. I am smiling for the first time in months. I will work through your workbook and will pass this on to anyone I know that fits the mold.

"Thank you so much for helping me. I look forward to reading more and learning everything you have to say on this subject."

~ E.C.

"I am now completely pain free after following your program... I am a skeptic by nature and had I not gone through this process myself, I wouldn't have ever believed it possible... When I get an occasional twinge of pain somewhere, I no longer worry that it will last or that it is a physical injury. How liberating to be free from worry about pain hereafter. So I am grateful to you for your great work. I wish there were more doctors like you. Thanks again."

~ J.T.

"I listened (to a podcast interview on "The Healthy Mind"), Dr. Schechter (nice hearing your voice again). The Workbook worked for Dr. Zafirides and it worked for me, too. Specifically (and immediately) it helped me deal with the untimely passing of my younger sister. And over time, getting things out of my head and into a journal helped me, as you articulated in the Podcast, "to write about emotions rather than obsessing about pain." The debilitating back pains I used to suffer from a couple of times a year? Gone. By keeping a journal, I realized the pain corresponded with dates that were especially meaningful to me. Since that realization—since acknowledging the emotional pain associated with those dates—zero back pain."

~ M.R.

"It has taken me awhile to write since it is hard to express my gratitude for all that you did for our son. He has returned to school and is majoring in engineering. After his first few days there, we received an excited phone call letting us know he played basketball (for the first time in almost two years). The joy in his voice was priceless. After only a month working with you, there was a distinct and dramatic improvement in his condition and mental outlook. He is more active and plans to play intramural sports. We believe that he has reclaimed his life and finally sees a future after a very difficult two years.

"We are very grateful for all you did for our son. We thank you for giving him back his life."

~ R. and T.

"Following an athletic and academic career at UCLA, in my early 20's I started to suffer with a variety of maladies. Among them was lower back pain and Crohn's disease. With my back, it began with years of low grade pain, but one day about 10 years ago, while going for a layup during a basketball game, I felt something pop and immediately hunched over in acute distress.

"Over the next 8 months I tried everything under the sun to get better, but I got worse and did less and less activity – including surfing. Once I hit rock bottom, a friend, who kept referring me to Dr. Sarno's work, convinced me to read the book "Healing Back Pain" – and my life changed from that point.

"Forcing myself to take Sarno's word on full faith, over the next few months I got progressively better – from about a 9 to 3 on the pain scale. Now believing that something special was going on, my same friend convinced me to visit Dr. Schechter to reinforce the diagnosis – and that is exactly what it did. After meeting with Dr. Schechter and doing his workbook a few times, my pain went from a 3 to a 1 and has since faded to 0.

"With an increased faith in my body, and a better understanding of my unique psychology, I applied similar principles to my Crohn's and was able to rid myself of this disorder entirely – without diet, medicine, or lifestyle.

"Since then about 5 years have passed and I continue my journey of self-discovery. I am a HUGE believer in Mind-Body medicine and do all I can to support its promotion. I just turned 40 and I am the happiest and healthiest I have ever been – thanks to bold, pioneering physicians like Sarno, Schechter, and others."

~ J.C.

"You may recall meeting with me earlier this year. I had been suffering from RSI (arm pain) for five years and severe GI issues for several months. You took one look at me and called TMS. You are the man!

"Following your referral to Alan G. and Daniel Lyman, I embarked on eight weeks of therapy and I'm proud to report I've made a full recovery. Full! GI issues---Gone. Arm issues---Gone.

"I'm back in the gym. I'm playing guitar. I'm typing. I'm texting. You name it! And one day when I have children I'm going to hold them high.

"Words cannot suffice for the debt of gratitude I owe to you. From the bottom of my heart, I thank you for the work you did with me and continue to do for others.

"And please forgive my handwriting. Some things even TMS therapy can't cure."

~ N. G.

CHAPTER XIV

Summary and Take Home Lessons

You are coming to the end of this book. You may have started reading this book due to your own pain, or that of a loved one. I trust you have learned a lot along the way.

Let's recap:

A person with pain usually gets better. For example, much back pain resolves in a week. Most back pain is gone in six weeks. Other painful conditions resolve in days to a few weeks, rarely a month.

If your pain persists, it is called chronic pain, and your pain in the mind/brain is going through a chronification process. It is changing and shifting and becoming more painful due to your brain and emotions, and less due to the original injury or trauma that triggered it. Maybe nothing physical triggered the pain at all. It was always a mind-body syndrome and it became more solidified after a few months.

We have learned in this book about the types of pain, the types of personality factors that can solidify and entrench pain, and the early evidence from Dr. John Sarno of a phenomenon we refer to as TMS.

TMS is that process and diagnosis by which physical pain is really re-understood to be a mind/brain process with a huge emotional input. It is reversible with the right treatment. I have reviewed the evidence with you for this phenomenon, both clinical research results and the brain science of fMRI imaging.

I have laid out how I make this diagnosis and what I advise my patients with this diagnosis to do, starting with reading and journaling. I have discussed the key elements of a home program and described in detail the Twelve Stages of Healing. I have discussed the crucial Seven Lessons of Pain that may have shaken up your notions of what pain is and where it comes from.

The following chapters review more research in this field. I explain to doctors and health care practitioners how they can understand and utilize this information in their own practices. I have shared many inspiring case studies and even more gratifying testimonials of success from real people that I have treated.

I finish off with recommendations for further study, such as The MindBody Workbook, the home program that I have developed, books and materials by other experts in this field. I have discussed the important role of psychotherapy, for some people with this condition, and described how to find a good practitioner in your area or how to utilize the telephone, SKYPE or FaceTime to connect to regional or national experts in the emotional side of this disorder.

I have included terms and definitions to learn more of the language that we use in this field. I believe that I have left you with hope and a way to move forward.

PAIN IS REAL

Your mind/brain, your nervous system and your emotions are very real. By and large, doctors have focused too much on the physical and not enough on the psychological, the mind/brain and the nervous system. They miss the key area of where the pain comes from, why it lasts and how to get rid of it.

In this book, I have reviewed the reasons why treatment for pain is often unsuccessful. I described a research-tested approach to chronic pain that successfully empowers the individual with pain.

Chapter XIV, Summary and Take Home Lessons

The approach works top-down, from brain to body, not vice-versa. The model builds upon the pioneering work of John E. Sarno, M.D., and my own 25 years of experience in this field.

The method of healing requires some work. Most things that are worthwhile do. Based upon my experience, this program is easily doable by people of all ages and backgrounds. Most helpful is an open mind and a willing spirit. It is a learning process, a change in the software of your brain that fixes what you thought was bad hardware in your body.

A SOFTBALL STORY, THE TMS WAY

I will finish with a story that I tell patients. It illustrates the difference between TMS pain and ordinary suffering. It describes the difference between a TMS-prone person and other folks.

Think about softball. Maybe you have played this game at one time or another. It is a great game, but it combines an ideal muscle tightness and soreness experiment. Sit a lot. Stand still for a while. Then run at full speed to a base or to catch a ball.

If you have played softball after the age of 20, here is what you can expect:

You play Sunday and have a good time. On Monday morning, you are a little stiff. On Tuesday, you are more stiff and walking a bit slowly. By Wednesday, it is a little better. By Thursday, a lot better and by Friday you forgot you played softball.

Here is a TMS response to this sport: You play on Sunday and enjoy it. On Monday, you are stiff. Tuesday, you are more stiff and starting to worry a little. Wednesday, you are really stiff and worrying a lot, wondering if you are injured or whether you have suffered semi-permanent damage. By Thursday, you are in bed and by Friday you are calling the doctor.

Hopefully with this book, you will reduce the worry, avoid the bed rest and not need to see your doctor. At least after softball.

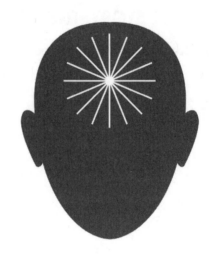

GLOSSARY

Definition of Terms

Acute - of short duration, typically less than six weeks

Acupuncture - a form of Chinese medicine in which a practitioner utilizes needles and herbs to affect energy in the body (chi) and treats health conditions including pain

Amplification - a process in the nervous system whereby pain signals are made "louder" or more powerful; the opposite of a calming effect. Believed to originate in the brain and efferent fibers down through the spinal cord

Anterior Cingulate Gyrus - a brain region also important to pain processing

Benign - not harmful; not serious

Cartesian Duality - mind and matter are different things that can affect one another; this philosophy is often blamed for the difficulty modern science and medicine has had with integrating mind and body (derived from Rene Descartes.)

Catastrophizing - the tendency to think the worst about a health situation, to amplify worry and consider a relatively minor issue a castastrophe

Chronic - of long duration, more than 6 months (3 months in some studies)

Chiropractor - a doctor whose approach to the musculoskeletal system is to focus primarily on alignment of the spine; a discipline that emphasizes structural spinal changes, some subtle, as the root of much back pain (and other illnesses). The field does however include very skilled and dedicated practitioners closer to physical therapists and also those who emphasize neurological and emotional adjustments as well.

Chronification - the process of an acute condition moving toward a chronic state, the transition between the two

Controlled - a study with a control group

Control Group - a group of participants in a study who are not given the active treatment intervention; a comparison group to the actively treated group

Diabetic Neuropathy - a condition among diabetes where the sensory nerves do not function as well as they should and the patient feels less in, e.g. the foot

Disc - a gelatinous or fibrous structure between the bones in the spine

Discogram - a moderately painful test where dye is injected into one or more spinal discs and the patient is asked if the injection reproduces the usual pain. A "positive" test is one where the patient says, "Yes, that is my usual pain." Studies suggest the test is not that reliable.

Descartes - a French philosopher, mathematician and writer, lived mostly in Holland and wrote about the mind in the 17th century ("I think therefore I am.")

DPS: Distraction Pain Syndrome - a name that emphasizes the role of distraction in the chronic pain that occurs from emotional factors

Dysautonomia - hereditary condition of altered function in the autonomic nervous system affecting digestion, vomiting, sensation, etc.

Efferent nerve signals - come from the brain to the body. While the motor signals are well known and allow us to move, sensory inhibitory and amplifying signals have also been identified, explaining the modulation of the pain experience by the brain; opposite of afferent signals that go to the brain

Ego - per Freud the organized realistic part that mediates between the id and superego

Endorphins and Enkephalins - naturally existing brain chemicals that appear to provide pain relief, mood elevation, etc.

ERCP: Endoscopic Retrograde Cholangio-Pancreatography - a procedure that looks at the common bile duct, pancreas, etc. through a tube inserted through the mouth down the throat, stomach, etc.

Flare-Up - re-occurrence of a condition that has improved or resolved

fMRI: Functional MRI - an MRI (Magnetic Resonance Imaging) scan that measures function, not just structure; this is not what you have had on your knee

Freud - founder of psychology, psychoanalysis and the physician who described the unconscious as a construct

Guarding - restriction of movement that occurs in people with chronic pain and other conditions; a reaction to pain that can become entrenched in the nervous system

Herniated Disc - a structural lesion where a soft structure between the bones in the back protrudes; may touch a nerve or irritate one; also may be completely without symptoms

Id - per Freud the primitive, emotional part of the mind

Irritable Bowel Syndrome - sensitive digestive tract that manifests as frequent diarrhea or constipation or alternating symptoms; not due to infection or inflammation

Metastatic Cancer - cancer that has spread away from its original location

Mind/Brain - a way of describing the reality of the mind and the closeness between brain and mind; mind as embodied in brain; brain as physical manifestation of mind

Mind-Body - the important linkage between our central nervous system, our controlling neural processes and the rest of the body (aka MindBody)

Myofascial - the muscle and fascia of the body; a common location for soft tissue injuries of back, neck, etc.; also "Myofascial pain"

Osteomyelitis - infection in the bone that is typically treated with intravenous antibiotics for an extended period of time

Pain Psychologist - a psychologist (typically Ph.D. or Psy.D.) who treats pain, often with a behavioral approach, with a goal of helping patients to manage a painful disorder

Phantom Limb Pain - the phenomenon where a person feels pain coming from an arm or leg that has been partially or totally amputated

Piriformis - a muscle in the buttocks adjacent to the sciatic nerve

PPD - Psycho-Physiological Disorder, from the medical words for mind-body

Pre Frontal Cortex - an area of the brain involved in processing higher level thought, attention, and pain

Psychosomatic - another medical word for mind-body; a real physical condition whose root may be in the mind/brain (psyche—mind/emotions; soma—body)

Psychophysiological - a medical word that says the same thing

Randomized - a study where participants are randomly assigned to different treatment groups or non-treatment or delayed treatment. By doing so randomly, each group should be similar to one another.

Reductionism - a complex system broken down to its parts; an approach to studying and understanding things by breaking them down; criticism is that something is lost about the overall system in the breaking down

Sarno: John E. Sarno, M.D. - pioneer of mind-body medicine; coined the diagnosis TMS; clinician and author of four popular books on TMS pain as well as many journal articles (in other subjects as well); retired 2012

Sensory Stimulus - sensations in the body that alert the mind to something of potential importance

Somatize - somatic means related to the body; somatize is to express emotions in a physical way

Spine Surgeon - an orthopedist or neurosurgeon who specializes in the treatment of spinal disorders by surgery

Sub-Acute - a condition lasting more than the acute period (e.g. 6 weeks) and not as long as the chronic period (e.g. 3-6 months)

Superego - per Freud the civilized controlling part of the mind

Tender Points - areas on the back that are often tender in people with TMS; overlap with, but fewer than, and different from the fibromyalgia tender points

Thecal - thecal sac is the sac around the spinal cord

TMS: Tension Myoneural Syndrome - pain syndrome caused by emotional issues and central nervous system pathways; mind/brain phenomenon with real pain; the mindbody syndrome

TMS Psychotherapist - a therapist, LCSW, MFT, Ph.D., etc.; with additional training and expertise and a focus on treating painful and functional disorders from a mind-body perspective utilizing the

TMS model

ADDITIONAL NOTE: COSTS OF PAIN TO SOCIETY

1) Institute of Medicine of the National Academies Report. "Relieving Pain in America: A Blueprint for Transforming Prevention, Care, Education, and Research," 2011. (Page 260) The National Academies Press, Washington DC.

2) Stewart, et al, JAMA 2003; 290: 2443.

Pain results in lost productivity of U.S. workers between $297.4 billion to $335.5 billion in 2010, according to the Institute of Medicine. Roughly 4% of the cost came from lost days of work, 29% from hours of lost work and 67% from lower wages. (1)

Another study looked again at the cost of pain to the U.S. economy and came up with $61.2 billion in lost productivity a year in the early 2000s, according to a study by Walter "Buzz" Stewart, Ph.D., MPH, in the Journal of the American Medical Association. That figure did not include any health care and disability payments. (2) These are all very large numbers.

Clearly, pain is a big problem for the economy. More importantly, it is a huge issue for you, the sufferer.

REFERENCES

CHAPTER I

1) Bigos S, Bowyer O, Braen G, et al. Acute low back problems in adults. Clinical Practice Guideline. Quick Reference Guide Number 14. Rockville, MD: US Department of Health and Human Services, Public Health Service, Agency for Health Care Policy and Research, AHCPR Pub. No. 95-0643. December 1994. (AHCPR Consensus Guidelines)

2) Cherkin, D. , Deyo R., et al A Comparison of Physical Therapy, Chiropractic, and an Educational Booklet, N Engl J Med 1998; 339:1021-1029.

3) Malmivaara, A., et al The Treatment of Low Back Pain. NEJM 1995 332: 351-5.

4) Linton, S., et al. Early Intervention. Pain 1993; 54:353-9.

5) CDC (Center for Disease Control), reported by Nadia Kounang, CNN News Source, May 2014.

6) Mafi, John N.; McCarthy, Ellen P. Ph.D.,; Davis, Roger B. Worsening Trends in the Management and Treatment of Back Pain. JAMA Intern Med. 2013; 173(17):1573-1581.

7) Schofferman, J. et al, Childhood psychological trauma correlates with unsuccessful lumbar spine surgery. Spine 1992 Jun; 17(6 Suppl):S138-44..

8) Weinstein JN, et al. (2006). Surgical vs non-operative treat-

ment for lumbar disk herniation: The spine patient outcomes research trial (SPORT): A randomized trial. JAMA, 296(20): 2441–2450.

9) Schechter, D. and Smith, A., Distraction Pain Syndrome, Evidence Based Integrative Medicine, 2006.

10) PPDA www.ppda.org

11) Schechter, D., Smith, A., et al, Outcomes of a Mind-Body Treatment Program for Chronic Back Pain with No Distinct Structural Pathology: A Case Series of Patients Diagnosed and Treated as Tension Myositis Syndrome. Alternative Therapies, Vol. 13, No. 5, Sept/Oct 2007.

12) Schechter, D. The MindBody Workbook. MindBody Medicine Publications, 1999.

13) Schechter, D. The MindBody Patient Panel, MindBody Medicine Publications 2004.

14) Schechter, D. The MindBody Audio Program, MindBody Medicine Publications.

CHAPTER II

1) http://en.wikipedia.org/wiki/Congenital_insensitivity_to_pain_with_anhidrosis

2) Turk and Wilson, Fear of Pain as a Prognostic Factor in Chronic Pain. Current Pain Headache Rep. April 2010, 14(2) 88-95.

3) Cherkin DC, Deyo RA, Wheeler K, et al. Physicians' views about treating low back pain: the results of national survey. Spine 1995; 20:1.

4) Hashmi JA1, Baliki MN, et al and Apkarian AV. Shape shifting pain: chronification of back pain shifts brain representation from nociceptive to emotional circuits. Brain. 2013 Sep; 136(Pt 9):2751-68.

5) Cignacco, EL, et al. Oral sucrose for pain relief in preterms. *Pediatrics*, Vol. 129 No. 2 February 1, 2012 pp. 299 -308.

6) Cain, et al, Discover Biology, Norton and Company, 2006; online animation --http://www.sumanasinc.com/webcontent/animations/content/reflexarcs.html

7) Nikolajsen, L, and Jensen, TS. Phantom Limb Pain. British Journal of Anaesthesia; vol 87, no. 1, 107-116, 2001.

8) Ramachandran, V. S.; Hirstein, William The Perception of Phantom Limbs: The D. O. Hebb Lecture. Brain 121 (1): 1603-1630, 2008,.

9) Flor, H Phantom limb pain: characteristics, causes and treatment. Lancet, 1, 182-189(2002).

10) Beecher, HK. The Pain in Men Wounded in Battle. Annals of Surgery, January, 1946.

11) Leuchter, AF, et al. Changes in Brain Function of Depressed Subjects. Am J. Psychiatry 159:122-129, January 2002.

12) Keltner, JR, Fields, HR, et al. Isolating the Modulatory Effect of Expectation on Pain Transmission: A Functional Magnetic Resonance Imaging Study. The Journal of Neuroscience, April 19, 2006, 26(16):4437-4443.

CHAPTER III

1) http://goalistics.com/2011/04/coping-pain-catastrophic-thinking-pain-worse/

2) Ghazizadeh A, Ambroggi F, Odean N, Fields HL. Prefrontal cortex mediates extinction of responding by two distinct neural mechanisms in accumbens shell. J Neurosci. 2012 Jan 11; 32(2):726-37.

3) Oxford Dictionaries, Online Edition.

4) Sarno, JE, Mind Over Back Pain. William Morrow & Co., New York, 1984.

5) Sarno, JE, Healing Back Pain. Warner Books, New York, 1991.

6) Sarno, J. E., The Mindbody Prescription. Warner Books, New York, 1998.

7) Sarno, JE, The Divided Mind. Regan Books, New York, 2006.

8) http://specularimage.wordpress.com/2011/04/07/the-triune-brain-meets-the-id-ego-and-super-ego/

9) Solms, Mark. Freud Returns. Scientific American, May 2004, P. 84-89.

10) Schechter ,D and Smith, A. et al. Back Pain as a distraction pain syndrome: A Window to a Whole New Dynamic in Integrative Medicine. Evidence Based Integrative Medicine, Vol. 2, No. 1, p. 3-8, 2005.

11) http://www.chop.edu/service/amplified-musculoskeletal-pain-syndrome/about-amps/amps-recurrence-prevention.html

12) Bigos, S., Battie, M., et al. A Prospective Study of work Perceptions and psychosocial factors affecting the report of back injury. Spine 1991, June 16(6) 688.

13) Friedman and Rosenman, Type A Behavior and Your Heart, Knopf, March 12, 1974.

14) Friedman and Rosenman, op cit.

CHAPTER IV

1) Jensen, M., Brant-Zawadzki, M., Obuchowski, N., MRI of the Lumbar Spine in People Without Back Pain, N Engl J Med 1994;

331:69-74.

2) Chou R, Qaseem A, Snow V, Casey D, Cross JT Jr, Shekelle P, Owens DK; Diagnosis and treatment of low back pain: a joint clinical practice guideline from the American College of Physicians and the American Pain Society. Clinical Efficacy Assessment Subcommittee of the American College of Physicians; American College of Physicians; American Pain Society Low Back Pain Guidelines Panel. Ann Intern Med. 2007 Oct 2; 147(7):478-91.

3) Kuhn, Thomas. The Structure of Scientific Revolutions, 2nd edition. University of Chicago Press, 1970.

4) Lemoine, N., The clinician-scientist: a rare breed under threat in a hostile environment Dis Model Mech. 2008 Jul-Aug; 1(1): 12–14.

5) Smith, A., HMOs Would Be Wise To Investigate Alternative Ways To Improve Health. Managed Care. Jan. 2004.

6) Schechter, D. "TMS Questionnaire." First Published on www.mindbodymedicine.com, approx. 1999.

CHAPTER V

1) Sarno, JE, Mind Over Back Pain. William Morrow & Co., New York, 1984.

2) Solms, Mark. Freud Returns. Scientific American, May 2004, P. 84-89.

3) http://www.n-psa.org/

4) LeDoux, Joseph. The Emotional Brain: The Mysterious Underpinnings of Emotional Life. New York: Simon & Schuster, 1996.

5) Ramachandran, VS.Consciousness and Cognition. 4: 22-51, 1995

CHAPTER VI

1) Vastag, B. Scientists find connections in the brain between emotional and physical pain. JAMA Nov. 12 2003 vol. 290 no 18, p 2389.

2) Kirmayer LJ, Robbins JM, Dworkind M, et al. Somatization and the recognition of depression and anxiety in primary care. Am J Psychiatry 1993;150:734-741

3) Holroyd, KA, et al. Management of Chronic Tension Type Headache with tricyclic antidepressant medication, stress management therapy, and their combination: a randomized controlled trial. JAMA 2001: 285: 2208-2215.

4) Stahl, a psycho-pharmacologist UCSD from JAMA Nov 12, 2003 interviewed in Medical News and Perspectives.

5) Eisenberger, N. Lieberman, M., and Williams, K. Does Rejection Hurt? An fMRI Study of Social Exclusion. Science 2003: 302:290-92, Oct. 2003 and others.

6) Derbyshire, s et al. Cerebral Activation During Hypnotically Induced and Imagined Pain. NeuroImage, 2004, 23: 392-401.

7) Kong, et al. Functional connectivity of the frontoparietal network predicts cognitive modulation of pain. Pain 154(3): 459-467, 2013.

8) https://www.rheumatology.org/Practice/Clinical/Patients/Diseases_And_Conditions/Back_Pain/ Brain. 2013 Sept; 136 (Pt 9) 2751-68. Hashmi, et al).

9) Bantick, SJet al. Imaging how attention modulates pain in humans using functional MRI. Brain (2002) 125 (2): 310-319.

10) Hadler, NM. MRI for regional back pain. Less MRI, better understanding. JAMA 2003; 289 (21) 2863-4.

11) Interview with Dr. Pohl, July 30, 2012, in Psychology Today.

12) Coste J, et al. Prognosis and Quality of Life in Acute Low Back Pain. Arthritis Care and Research, 2004; 51 (2) 168-76.

13) Power, C, et al. Predictors of Low Back Pain Onset in a Prospective British Study. Am J Public Health 2001; 91: 1671-78.

14) Lemos, AT, et al. Low back pain and associated factors in children and adolescents in a private school in Southern Brazil. Cad Saude Publica. 2013 Nov; 29(11):2177-85.

15) Biggs, AM, et al. Effect of childhood adversity on health related quality of life in patients with upper abdominal or chest pain. Gut. Feb 2004; 53(2): 180–186.

16) Schofferman, J. et al, Childhood psychological trauma correlates with unsuccessful lumbar spine surgery. Spine 1992 Jun; 17(6 Suppl):S138-44.

17) Moseley, L. Widespread brain activity during an abdominal task markedly reduced after pain physiology education: fMRI evaluation of a single patient with chronic low back pain. Australian J Physiotherapy 2005, vol 51, p. 48-52.

18) Bell, K & Meadows, E. Efficacy of a brief relaxation training intervention for pediatric recurrent abdominal pain. Cognitive and Behavioral Practice 20(1): 81-92. 2013.

19) Van Korff, M et al. Chronic spinal pain and physical mental comorbidity. Pain, 2005; 113:33-9.

20) Croft, The Back Letter. Feb. 2005.

21) Maeda, F. et al. Thinking as a Prescription for Pain Relief. Bone and Joint, Vol. 10, No.6, June 2004.

22) Smyth, JM et al, Effects of writing about stressful experiences on symptom reduction in patients with asthma or rheumatoid arthritis: A Randomized Trial. JAMA 1999; 281: 1304-09.

23) Vincent NK, Walker JR. Perfectionism and chronic insom-

nia. J Psychosom Res. 2000 Nov; 49(5):349-54.

24) Flett, GL, et al. Perfectionism, psychosocial impact and coping with irritable bowel disease: A study of patients with Crohn's disease and ulcerative colitis. J Health Psychol May 2011 16: 561-571, first published on February 23, 2011.

25) Turk, DC and Wilson, H. Fear of pain as a prognostic factor in chronic pain: conceptual models, assessment, and treatment implications. Curr Pain Headache Rep. 2010 Apr; 14(2):88-95.

26) Schneider, DL, et al. Arthritic Changes on Xrays Generally Have Little Functional Significance. J Bone and Joint Surgery, 1994; 72-A3; 403-408.

27) Boden, S. Abnormal MRI scans of the Lumbar spine in asymptomatic subjects. A Prospective Study. J Bone Joint Surgery Am. 1990. 72: 403-408.

28) Jensen, M., Brant-Zawadzki, M., Obuchowski, N., MRI of the Lumbar Spine in People Without Back Pain, N Engl J Med 1994; 331:69-74.

29) Carragee, Eugene. Are first-time episodes of serious LBP associated with new MRI findings? The Spine Journal, Vol. 6, No. 6, Nov 2006, p 624-35.

CHAPTER VII

These patient stories are, as described earlier, patients of mine for whom demographic details, gender, age and occupation, have been scrambled enough to anonymize them while retaining the essence of their condition and recovery for illustrative purposes.

CHAPTER VIII

The TMS Questionnaire was first published online by David

Schechter, M.D., ca. 1996 and has been utilized in his office and in his written materials since then. The Questionnaire is a copyrighted work, all rights reserved.

CHAPTER IX

1) Schechter, D., The MindBody Workbook. MindBody Medicine Publications, 1999.

2) Pennebaker JW, Beall SK. A. "Confronting a traumatic event: toward an understanding of inhibition and disease." Journal of Abnormal Psychology. 95: 274-81.

3) Baikie, K and Wilhelm, H. Emotional and Physical Health Benefits of Expressive Writing. Advances in Psychiatric Treatment Advances in Psychiatric Treatment 11: 338-346. 2005.

4) Zauszniewski JA et al, Res Nurs Health 2014 Feb 26;37(1):42-52.

5) Savoy, C., & Beitel, P. (1996). Mental imagery for basketball. International Journal of Sport Psychology, 27, 454-462.

6) Nicholson, R. et al, Psychological Risk Factors in Headache. Headache, March 2007, p. 413-426) 8- 22.

7) Mehling, W. Krause, J. Are difficulties in perceiving and expressing emotions associated with low back pain. Psychosomatic Research 58 (2005) 73-81

8) Parker, JDA Taylor RM, and Bagby, GJ. Toronto Alexithymia Scale. Journal of Psychosomatic Research 55 (2003) 269 – 275.

9) Creswell, C, and Chalder, T. Defensive Coping Styles in Chronic Fatigue Syndrome. J Psychosom Res 2001; 51: 607-10.

CHAPTER X

1) Malmivaara, A., et al The Treatment of Low Back Pain. NEJM 1995 332: 351-5.

2) Schechter, D. The MindBody Audio Program, MindBody Medicine Publications.

3) http://www.sparkpeople.com/mypage_public_journal_individual.asp?blog_id=4465850

CHAPTER XI

1) Schechter, D, At Home Educational Materials for Chronic Pain. Practical Pain Management, May/June 2004.

2) Schechter, D. and Smith, A. Psychosomatic Medicine, Vol. 67, No.1, online, p. A-101.

3) Schechter ,D and Smith, A. et al. Back Pain as a distraction pain syndrome: A Window to a Whole New Dynamic in Integrative Medicine. Evidence Based Integrative Medicine, Vol. 2, No. 1, p. 3-8, 2005.

4) Schechter, D. et al, Outcomes of a Mind-Body Healing Program for Chronic Back Pain with No Distinct Structural Pathology: A Case Series of Patients Diagnosed and Treated as Tension Myositis Syndrome (TMS). Alternative Therapies in Health and Medicine; Sept/Oct. 2007.

5) Sarno JE, Etiology of neck and back pain as an autonomic myoneuralgia. Journal Of Nervous & Mental Disease: 55-59, 1981.

6) Sarno, JE, Psychosomatic Backache, Journal of Family Practice, 1977 Sep; 5(3):353-357,.

7) Rashbaum, I. and Sarno, JE. Psychosomatic Concepts in Chronic Pain. Archives Phys Med Rehab, 2003. Mar; 84 (3 Suppl 1) S76-80.

8) Coen, SJ, and Sarno, JE, J Am Acad Psychoanalysis. 1989 Fall;17(3):359-76.

9) Sarno, JE, Mind Over Back Pain. William Morrow & Co., New York, 1984.

10) Sarno, JE, Healing Back Pain. Warner Books, New York, 1991.

11) Sarno, JE, The Mindbody Prescription. Warner Books, New York, 1998.

12) Sarno, JE, The Divided Mind. Regan Books, New York, 2006.

13) Lumley MA1, Cohen JL, Borszcz GS, Cano A, Radcliffe AM, Porter LS, Schubiner H, Keefe FJ. Pain and Emotion, A Biopsychosocial Review. J Clin Psychol. 2011 Sep;67(9):942-68. doi: 10.1002/jclp.20816. Epub 2011 Jun 6.

14) Hsu MC, Schubiner H, Lumley MA, Stracks JS, Clauw DJ, Williams DA. J Gen Sustained Pain Reduction Through Affective Self-Awareness in Fibromyalgia. Intern Med. 2010 Oct;25(10):1064-70.

15) Hsu, MC, Schubiner, H. Recovery From Chronic Musculoskeletal Pain with Psychodynamic Consultation and Brief Intervention: Three Cases. Pain Med. 2010 Jun;11(6):977-80.

CHAPTER XII

1) Kirmayer LJ, Robbins JM, Dworkind M, et al. Somatization and the recognition of depression and anxiety in primary care. Am J Psychiatry 1993; 150:734-741.

CHAPTER XIII

1) Sarno, JE, Mind Over back Pain, William Morrow & Co., New York, 1984.

2) Sarno, JE, Healing Back Pain, Warner Books, New York, 1991.

3) Sarno, JE, The Mindbody Prescription. Warner Books, New York, 1998.

4) Sarno, JE, The Divided Mind, Regan Books, New York, 2006.

5) Schechter, D. The MindBody Workbook. MindBody Medicine Publications, 1999.

6) Schechter, D. The MindBody Patient Panel, MindBody Medicine Publications 2004.

7) Schechter, D. The MindBody Audio Program, MindBody Medicine Publications.

APPENDIX A
Resources

Books and Other Materials

John Sarno, M.D. 4 books (Chapter XIII: 1,2,3,4)

David Schechter, M.D.

> TMS Home Program consists of:
>
> The MindBody Workbook, Audio and DVD programs (References: Chapter XIII: 5, 6, 7)
>
> Website: www.MindBodyMedicine.com
>
> Research: www.smi-MindBodyResearch.org

Howard Schubiner, M.D. *Unlearn Your Pain*

David Hanscom, M.D. *Back In Control*

TMS wiki www.TMSwiki.org

Peter Zafirides, M.D. *The Healthy Mind Podcast*

> www.TheHealthyMind.com

Marc Sopher, M.D. *To Be or Not To Be Pain Free*

Nancy Selfridge, M.D. *Freedom From Fibromyalgia*

David Clarke, M.D. *They Can't Find Anything Wrong*

Partial List of Leading TMS Doctors

Ira Rashbaum, M.D., Rusk Institute, New York City, New York

Howard Schubiner, M.D., Providence Hospital, Southfield, Michigan

David Hanscom, M.D. and team, Swedish Hospital, Seattle, Washington

Marc Sopher, M.D., Exeter, New Hampshire

Peter Zafirides, M.D., Columbus, Ohio

Andrea Leonard-Segal, M.D., George Washington University Medical Center, Washington, D.C.

Along with a growing number of others, see:
www.mindbodymedicine.com/doctors.html or tms wiki website

Leading Psychotherapists

New York: Eric Sherman, Fran Anderson, Liz Wallenstein, others

Los Angeles: Alan Gordon, Arnold Bloch, Jill Solomon, Colleen Perry, Jessica Oifer; The Pain Psychology Center (Alan Gordon, Derek Sapico, and team), others

Australia: James Alexander

Leading Advocacy

Dave Clarke, M.D., PPDA

Rob Munger: TMS wiki

Other books:

The Open Focus Brain, Jim Robbins

The Talent Code, Daniel Coyle

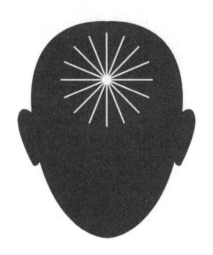

APPENDIX B

Dr. Schechter's Credentials

- Princeton University, Biochemistry, Senior Thesis Nucleotide Bonding

- New York University School of Medicine, Summer Research TMS with Sarno

- UCLA/Santa Monica Hospital Residency in Family Medicine

- Board Certified in Family Medicine and re-certified three additional times

- Faculty, USC/California Hospital Residency Program

- Assistant Clinical then Associate Clinical Professor, USC School of Medicine

- Board Certified (Certificate of Added Qualifications, CAQ) Sports Medicine, recertified two additional times

- USC/California Hospital Residency Program Faculty, Two Teaching Awards

- Lecturer: Over 100 lectures to physicians, residents, and medical students

- Creator of www.MindBodyMedicine.com; first website devoted to TMS

- Author of The MindBody Workbook

- Creator of The MindBody AudioProgram (set of three CD's)

- Host of The MindBody Patient Panel (DVD), 75 minutes)

- Podcasts on TMS and mind-body issues

- Guest on Television News, Radio Shows, Podcasts on TMS and other subjects

- Principal Investigator, Seligman Medical Institute 2003-2007

- Author of Peer-Reviewed articles on TMS in several journals

- Staff Physician, Cedars Sinai Medical Center

- Private Practice of Medicine, Beverly Hills and Culver City, California

- Credentialed Pain Practitioner, American Academy of Pain Management

- Top Doctor, Castle Connolly Directory, 2003- 2014

- Top Doctor, Men's Health Magazine, 2008

- Top Doctor, US News and World Report, 2011

- Husband and Father

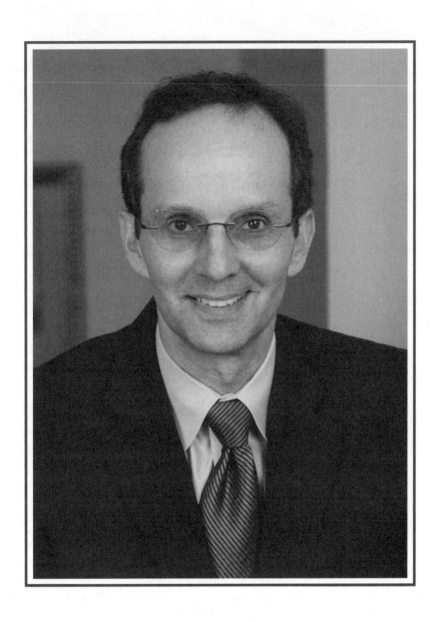

David Schechter, M.D.

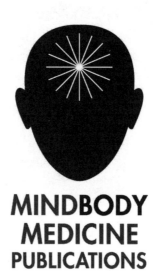

**MINDBODY
MEDICINE
PUBLICATIONS**

www.MindBodyMedicine.com